T0200314

Risk Factors for Posttraumatic Stress Disorder

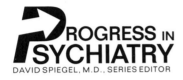

PROGRESS IN **PSYCHIATRY**

DAVID SPIEGEL, M.D., SERIES EDITOR

Number 58

Risk Factors for Posttraumatic Stress Disorder

Edited by
Rachel Yehuda, Ph.D.

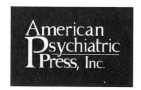

Washington, DC
London, England

Note: The authors have worked to ensure that all information in this book concerning drug dosages, schedules, and routes of administration is accurate as of the time of publication and consistent with standards set by the U.S. Food and Drug Administration and the general medical community. As medical research and practice advance, however, therapeutic standards may change. For this reason and because human and mechanical errors sometimes occur, we recommend that readers follow the advice of a physician who is directly involved in their care or in the care of a member of their family.

Copyright © 1999 American Psychiatric Press, Inc.
ALL RIGHTS RESERVED
Manufactured in the United States of America on acid-free paper
First Edition
02 01 00 99   4 3 2 1

American Psychiatric Press, Inc.
1400 K Street, N.W.
Washington, DC   20005
www.appi.org

Library of Congress Cataloging-in-Publication Data
Risk factors for posttraumatic stress disorder   /   edited by Rachel
    Yehuda. —   1st ed.
        p.   cm.   —   (Progress in psychiatry series   :   no. 58)
      Includes bibliographical references and index.
      1. Post-traumatic stress disorder—Risk factors. I. Yehuda, Rachel. II. Series.
      [DNLM: 1. Stress Disorders, Post-Traumatic—etiology. 2. Risk Factors.
    WM 170 R595 1999   /   W1 PR6781L no.58 1999]
    RC552.P67R57 1999
    616.85′21—dc21
    DNLM/DLC
    for Library of Congress   98-43412
                                                                                    CIP

British Library Cataloguing in Publication Data
A CIP record is available from the British Library.

Contents

Contributors

Naomi Breslau, Ph.D.
Director of Research, Department of Psychiatry, Henry Ford Health System, Detroit, Michigan; Professor, Department of Psychiatry, Case Western Reserve University School of Medicine, Cleveland, Ohio; Clinical Professor, Department of Psychiatry, University of Michigan School of Medicine, Ann Arbor, Michigan

Evelyn Bromet, Ph.D.
Professor, Department of Psychiatry and Behavioral Science, State University of New York at Stony Brook

Kathryn M. Connor, M.D.
Assistant Research Professor, Department of Psychiatry and Behavioral Sciences, Duke University Medical Center, Durham, North Carolina

Jonathan R. T. Davidson, M.D.
Professor, Department of Psychiatry and Behavioral Sciences; Director, Anxiety and Traumatic Stress Program, Duke University Medical Center, Durham, North Carolina

Matthew J. Friedman, M.D., Ph.D.
Executive Director, National Center for Post-traumatic Stress Disorder, White River Junction, Vermont; Professor of Psychiatry and Pharmacology, Dartmouth Medical School, Hanover, New Hampshire

Philip D. Harvey, Ph.D.
Professor of Psychiatry, Mount Sinai School of Medicine, New York, New York

Michael Hughes, Ph.D.
Professor, Department of Sociology, Virginia Polytechnic
Institute, Blacksburg, Virginia

Ronald C. Kessler, Ph.D.
Professor of Health Care Policy, Harvard Medical School,
Boston, Massachusetts

Michael J. Lyons, Ph.D.
Associate Professor, Boston University, Boston; Psychology
Department, Brockton VA Medical Center, Brockton,
Massachusetts

**A. C. McFarlane, M.D., F.R.A.N.Z.C.P., M.B.B.S.
(Dip.Psychother.)**
Professor and Head, Department of Psychiatry, University of
Adelaide, Australia

Christopher B. Nelson, Ph.D., M.P.H.
Scientist, World Health Organization, Division of Mental
Health & Prevention of Substance Abuse, Geneva, Switzerland

Scott P. Orr, Ph.D.
Research Psychologist, Department of Veterans Affairs,
Manchester, New Hampshire; Assistant Professor of
Psychology, Department of Psychiatry, Harvard Medical
School, Boston, Massachusetts

Roger K. Pitman, M.D.
Coordinator, Research and Development, Department of
Veterans Affairs, Manchester, New Hampshire; Associate
Professor of Psychiatry, Department of Psychiatry, Harvard
Medical School, Boston, Massachusetts

Paula P. Schnurr, Ph.D.
Deputy to the Executive Director, Department of Veterans Affairs, National Center for PTSD, White River Junction, Vermont; Research Associate Professor, Department of Psychiatry, Dartmouth Medical School, Hanover, New Hampshire

Arieh Y. Shalev, M.D.
Professor and Chairman, Department of Psychiatry; Director, Center for Traumatic Stress, Hadassah University Hospital, Jerusalem, Israel

Amanda Sonnega, Ph.D.
Research Investigator, Survey Research Center, University of Michigan, Ann Arbor

William R. True, Ph.D.
Professor of Community Health, School of Public Health, and Department of Psychiatry and Human Behavior, School of Medicine, St. Louis University Health Sciences Center; Research Service, St. Louis Veterans Affairs Medical Center, St. Louis, Missouri

Melanie J. Vielhauer, Ph.D.
Psychologist, Boston Veterans Affairs Outpatient Clinic, Boston, Massachusetts

Rachel Yehuda, Ph.D.
Director, Traumatic Stress Studies Program and Professor, Department of Psychiatry, Mount Sinai School of Medicine, Bronx VA Medical Center, Bronx, New York

Introduction to the *Progress in Psychiatry Series*

The Progress in Psychiatry Series is designed to capture in print the excitement that comes from assembling a diverse group of experts from various locations to examine in detail the newest information about a developing aspect of psychiatry. This series emerged as a collaboration between the American Psychiatric Association's (APA) Scientific Program Committee and the American Psychiatric Press, Inc. Great interest is generated by a number of the symposia presented each year at the APA annual meeting, and we realized that much of the information presented there, carefully assembled by people who are deeply immersed in a given area, would unfortunately not appear together in print. The symposia sessions at the annual meetings provide an unusual opportunity for experts who otherwise might not meet on the same platform to share their diverse viewpoints for a period of 3 hours. Some new themes are repeatedly reinforced and gain credence, whereas in other instances disagreements emerge, enabling the audience and now the reader to reach informed decisions about new directions in the field. The Progress in Psychiatry Series allows us to publish and capture some of the best of the symposia and thus provide an in-depth treatment of specific areas that might not otherwise be presented in broader review formats.

Psychiatry is, by nature, an interface discipline, combining the study of mind and brain, of individual and social environments, of the humane and the scientific. Therefore, progress in the field is rarely linear—it often comes from unexpected sources. Furthermore, new developments emerge from an array of viewpoints that do not necessarily provide immediate agreement but rather expert examination of the issues. We intend to present innovative ideas and data that will enable you, the reader, to participate in this process.

We believe the Progress in Psychiatry Series will provide you with an opportunity to review timely, new information in specific fields of interest as they are developing. We hope you find that the excitement of the presentations is captured in the written word and that this book proves to be informative and enjoyable reading.

David Spiegel, M.D.
Series Editor
Progress in Psychiatry Series

Introduction

Posttraumatic stress disorder (PTSD) can occur following exposure to extremely traumatic events. Recent estimates suggest that as many as 14% of the people in the United States develop this condition at some point in their lives. This makes PTSD an enormous public health problem. What has become clear in recent years, however, is that PTSD does not occur in everyone who is exposed to traumatic events. Thus, although exposure to trauma appears to be a necessary requirement of PTSD, the presence of a traumatic event does not sufficiently explain why PTSD develops or persists. This has led the authors in this volume to attempt to identify risk factors that may increase the likelihood of developing chronic disorder after exposure to trauma.

The new emphasis on risk factors for PTSD represents a shift from the original conceptions of this disorder presented in the *Diagnostic and Statistical Manual of Mental Disorders* that emphasized the importance of the traumatic event as the single etiologic agent in PTSD. Indeed, the main point of establishing the diagnosis of PTSD was to provide a psychiatric category that explained the presence of chronic symptoms after trauma exposure in otherwise "normal" individuals. The proponents of the diagnosis hoped that such a category would spare victims the indignity of being misunderstood as "neurotic" or constitutionally weak for succumbing to the effects of a traumatic event and would shift the emphasis of treatment from minimizing the impact of such traumatic events to exploring their significance.

The diminution of the impact of environmental stressors to psychiatric symptoms became particularly fashionable as neurobiological findings began to be applied to psychiatric research in the late 1960s and the 1970s. This research was largely interpreted as suggesting that psychiatric symptoms were not only biologically driven but also likely to be genetically determined. In 1980, against the backdrop of the increasing importance of genetics and neuroscience, it was courageous for the proponents of PTSD to reassert the importance of environmental events in the induction of any psychiatric illness.

One of the original intentions behind the diagnosis of PTSD was to define a traumatic stressor as an experience so objectively horrifying that most people would understand why there could be resultant symptoms. If every trauma survivor developed similar symptoms after exposure, this would have served as further validation of the hypothesis of PTSD, namely, that trauma resulted in posttraumatic symptoms. However, epidemiological studies of the prevalence of PTSD demonstrated that the objective characteristics of events were not sufficient predictors of this disorder. This led to a consideration of subjective characteristics, particularly of the personal appraisal of the event by the survivor. By focusing on both the objective characteristics of an event (i.e., as involving "actual or threatened death or serious injury or a threat to the physical integrity of self or others") and the subjective response of "fear, helplessness, or horror," DSM-IV implicitly acknowledged that there may be diversity in human responses to traumatic events. It also implied that emotional responses to even the most traumatic events cannot be assumed. However, DSM-IV did not explicitly address the issue of *why* some people would respond to trauma with fear, helplessness, or horror, whereas others would not. This issue is the focus of the current volume.

Putative risk factors for PTSD can be divided into two broad categories: those pertinent to the traumatic event (e.g., severity or type of trauma) and those relevant to individuals who experience the event (e.g., gender, prior experiences, or personality characteristics). Although some risk factors for PTSD appear to be related to prior experiences, data have also emerged implicating biological and, possibly, genetic risk factors for PTSD.

The information currently available about risk factors for PTSD has been derived largely through retrospective analysis of differences between trauma-exposed persons with and without PTSD. Historically, phenomenological and biological differences between trauma survivors with and without PTSD have been interpreted as reflecting consequences of the traumatic event or correlates of posttraumatic disorder. However, it is not unreasonable to consider the possibility that any differences between trauma survivors with and without PTSD might also reflect risk factors for the development of PTSD. It has become critical to determine strategies for distinguishing between predisposing and stress-related alterations in trauma survivors with PTSD. One such approach involves identifying populations that are at increased risk for trauma exposure or PTSD and evaluating the extent to which these individuals resemble trauma-exposed survivors with PTSD. These and other strategies for assessing risk for PTSD are described in Chapter 1 by Harvey and myself.

One way to begin the task of identifying individuals at risk for PTSD is to survey the normal population and establish the characteristics of those who are exposed to traumatic events and who subsequently develop PTSD. In Chapter 2, Kessler and colleagues discuss how epidemiological studies have identified several important demographic and environmental risk factors for the development of PTSD after exposure to a traumatic event. An intriguing observation of this group has been that exposure to any particular focal trauma is not the most important predictor of PTSD. Rather, cumulative stress and, in particular, a history of prior exposure to trauma emerge as very important risk factors for PTSD.

In Chapter 3, True and Lyons discuss how studies of monozygotic and dizygotic twins (discordant for combat trauma) from the Vietnam Veterans Twin Registry have demonstrated that as much as 30% of some PTSD symptoms appear to have a genetic basis. In Chapter 4, Davidson and Connor demonstrate a more subtle familial relationship by their findings of increased PTSD among those with a family history of psychopathology. In Chapter 5, I describe findings of an increased prevalence of PTSD among adult children of Holocaust survivors and suggest that children of trauma survivors with PTSD may constitute an important high-risk group.

In Chapter 5, I also describe neuroendocrine alterations in the children of Holocaust survivors and suggest that these alterations are similar to those observed in trauma survivors with PTSD. The observation that "at risk" children of Holocaust survivors show lower cortisol levels compared with a comparison group of demographically comparable subjects provides the first prospective demonstration of a biological alteration similar to PTSD in a high-risk group. However, there are other suggestions of neurobiological risk factors, as discussed in Chapter 6 by Orr and Pitman. These investigators consider several potential neurological and neurocognitive risk factors for PTSD, including lower IQ, differences in cognitive performance, and reduced hippocampal volume. Orr and Pitman make the point that any or all of the memory-related findings in PTSD might reflect preexisting vulnerabilities rather than consequences of trauma exposure. Similarly, in Chapter 7, Shalev discusses the possibility that psychophysiological alterations in PTSD may also be risk factors for this disorder rather than consequences of the traumatic event. Indeed, using a prospective, longitudinal design, Shalev and his colleagues have determined that some psychophysiological variables may indeed represent risk factors. For example, heart rate at the time of the trauma appears to predict the subsequent development of PTSD. Other psychophysiological alterations, such as the startle response, clearly only emerge over time. The importance of prospective, longitudinal studies is further discussed by McFarlane in Chapter 8. McFarlane describes how biological changes in the early aftermath of traumatic events, in contrast to psychological changes, might predict the subsequent development of PTSD. One of the more exciting findings presented in this chapter is that the cortisol responses in the immediate aftermath of a traumatic event may actually predict whether an individual will or will not develop a psychiatric condition and may also shed light on which condition will be developed. In Chapter 9, Schnurr and Vielhauer remind us that a wide variety of factors that have been related historically to both environmental and biological factors can be easily identified and considered as risk factors. They describe studies of pretrauma personality characteristics that are essential in helping to delineate the individual differences in the response to trauma. In so doing, these authors again raise the issue of the nature of risk factors.

One of the important points emphasized in this volume is that it is extremely difficult to ascertain the etiology of risk factors for PTSD. Even the most experiential of risk factors do not necessarily reflect "environmental" as opposed to "genetic" origins. For example, the risk factor of prior victimization would more likely be a purely environmental risk factor if trauma exposure (i.e., environmental events) were randomly distributed. But in fact, in addition to there being risk factors for the development of PTSD, there are risk factors for exposure to traumatic events, as discussed in Chapters 2 and 3. Other risk factors for PTSD, such as being female, are also ambiguous in terms of origin. Since being female is also a risk factor for sexual victimization, it is unclear whether the experiential component (i.e., different environmental experiences) is more relevant than the biological factors (i.e., hormonal differences).

The risk factors mentioned in Chapters 2, 6, and 9 concerning past histories of behavior or psychological problems and neurotic or antisocial personalities, as well as the cognitive risk factor of lower intelligence, are similarly ambiguous. It could be argued that these characteristics are manifestations of early life experiences, but at the same time they may reflect expressions of genetic diatheses. The argument works both ways. Abuse early in life might lead to avoidance, sociopathy, conduct disorder, and lower intelligence as a reflection of pretrauma-related cognitive impairments. On the other hand, these traits may constitute the type of biological vulnerabilities that make trauma survivors less likely to recover from the effects of adversity.

The extent to which any of the risk factors are indicative of truly biological or even genetic phenomena, as opposed to environmental ones, is not clear. Even twin studies are not necessarily indicative of genetic factors because of the large shared environment in families, as pointed out in Chapter 3. In particular, the vulnerability for developing PTSD in a trauma survivor who has lived with a chronically mentally ill family member may reflect genetics, experience, or some combination. As noted in Chapter 5, children of Holocaust survivors reported feeling chronically stressed from hearing stories about the Holocaust and feeling affected by the disability of their parents. Thus, the increased prevalence of PTSD in twins, parents, or children of trauma survivors (Chapters 3, 4, and 5, respectively) may reflect vulnerability owing to these experiences rather than to inherited genes. In the case of the children of

Holocaust survivors, however, even if the diathesis of PTSD were somehow "biologically transmitted," the diathesis would still be a consequence of the traumatic stress in the parent. Thus, even the most biological of explanations for vulnerability must at some point deal with the fact that a traumatic event has occurred.

In Chapter 10, Friedman provides an elegant synthesis of the other chapters in this book and comments on how the findings reported therein can ultimately advance the field of traumatology. The identification of risk factors for PTSD might have important future application in helping to identify and treat individuals at much earlier stages following a traumatic experience and even to reduce trauma exposure (e.g., due to combat, occupations such as law enforcement or firefighting) in vulnerable individuals.

One of the most useful applications of the study of risk factors is the application of this knowledge to understanding why some individuals develop symptoms to lower-magnitude events. Indeed, as summarized in Chapter 2, epidemiological studies have provided solid support for the idea that the severity of a traumatic event is one of the most salient risk factors for the subsequent development of PTSD. The dose-response relationship between severity of the trauma and the development of PTSD implies that vulnerability factors may be particularly important as one moves down along the spectrum of horror and catastrophe. Because there is a qualitative difference between being subjected to purposeful torture and being involved in a motor vehicle accident—even though both experiences may be associated with life threat and physical and psychological injury—vulnerability factors may be more relevant in the induction of PTSD in response to the latter (lower magnitude) trauma. One strategy for studying risk factors in the development of PTSD is to compare vulnerability factors in those experiencing high-magnitude responses to moderately severe versus extremely severe events.

Finally, if lower-magnitude traumatic events are more likely to lead to PTSD under conditions of increased vulnerability (as suggested in Chapter 5), then vulnerable individuals might show exaggerated responses to "subthreshold" stressful events—that is, events that would not classically be considered as traumatic

enough to cause PTSD. Thus, the study of risk factors will ultimately further our understanding of the potency of all potentially
stressful life events.

Rachel Yehuda, Ph.D.

Acknowledgments

I would like to thank all the authors for their very thoughtful contributions to this volume and for providing an unusual richness to their discussions of risk for PTSD. No group of colleagues could make editing a book so easy. I would also like to thank the Progress in Psychiatry Series Editor, David Spiegel, M.D., for his inspiration and insightful comments. My colleagues and staff at the Mount Sinai School of Medicine and Bronx Veterans Affairs Medical Center—Robert Levengood, M.D., Julia Golier, M.D., Douglas Gerber, M.S.W., Larry Ibisch, M.S.W., Robert Grossman, M.D., Cheryl Wong, M.D., Morton Siegel, M.D., Burt Rosen, M.D., Edith Laufer, Ph.D., Ren-kui Yang, Ph.D., Ling Song Guo, M.D., Ilana Breslau, Ph.D., Dan Aferiot, M.S.W., James Schmeidler, Ph.D., Abbie Elkin, B.A., Susan Dolan, B.A., Nikki Kalkines, B.A., and Carolyn Jjingo, B.A., and Phil Wise and Tony Mason—have been a wonderful source of wisdom and support.

Most important, I thank my husband, Mitch, and children, Daniel, Erica, and Rebecca, who have been patient, understanding, supportive, and very generous.

Chapter 1

Strategies to Study Risk for the Development of PTSD

Philip D. Harvey, Ph.D., and Rachel Yehuda, Ph.D.

osttraumatic stress disorder (PTSD) is a psychiatric condition that can occur in individuals who experience extremely stressful or traumatic life events. However, this disorder is not an inevitable outcome of exposure to such events. The development of PTSD following trauma exposure appears to be partially determined by the type and severity of the traumatic stressor. Indeed, certain traumatic events, such as rape and torture, are associated with higher prevalence rates of PTSD than are natural disasters or motor vehicle accidents (reviewed by Kessler and colleagues in Chapter 2 of this volume). However, even in the most traumatic of situations, many individuals do not appear to develop symptoms of PTSD (Breslau et al. 1991; Davidson et al. 1991; Helzer et al. 1987). Furthermore, among those who develop symptoms in the immediate aftermath of traumatic events, only some will show signs of chronic PTSD (McFarlane 1992; Rothbaum et al. 1992). For this reason, it has recently been hypothesized that the development of chronic PTSD results from a combination of factors, only some of which are directly related to trauma exposure (Yehuda and McFarlane 1995).

One possible reason for the disparity between the prevalence of trauma (an objective fact) and the prevalence of PTSD (a subjective

Some of the work reported in this chapter was supported by grants from the National Institute of Mental Health (NIMH 49536, NIMH-59555 to R.Y.) and the Department of Veterans Affairs (VA Merit Award to R.Y.).

1

response) is that there is considerable individual variation in the perception of what is "traumatic" or distressing. A major question that has arisen in trying to understand the nature of PTSD is whether traumatic events are to be defined on the basis of the objective characteristics of the event or, rather, the individual's personal response of danger, terror, and/or helplessness. The initial intent of the diagnosis of PTSD was to consider the consequences of events that most people would find catastrophic and, as such, to relieve victims of the burden of feeling weak for succumbing to the effects of the traumatic event (Yehuda and McFarlane 1995). Thus, the focus of the diagnosis of PTSD was originally on the objective characteristics of the event that would, almost by definition, lead to impairment. However, it soon became clear that some individuals exposed to even the most traumatic events do not develop symptoms of PTSD. The failure to develop such symptoms is likely the result of subjective perceptions at the time of or subsequent to the event and not the impotence of the stressor. For example, it is possible that if an individual experiences a life-threatening situation without feeling an internal loss of control, and, in fact, perceives a mastery over the event by the very fact of his or her survival, then this person may feel triumphant, invigorated, or even invincible rather than victimized and vulnerable.

DSM-IV (American Psychiatric Association 1994) focuses on both the objective characteristics of an event (i.e., a traumatic event is defined as involving "actual or threatened death or serious injury, or a threat to the physical integrity of self or others") and the subjective response of the person exposed to the trauma ("fear, helplessness, or horror") (Table 1–1). However, DSM-IV does not explicitly address why some people respond to trauma with fear, helplessness, or horror whereas others do not.

In this chapter, we address the complex interaction of objective and subjective vulnerabilities to factors that might give rise to PTSD. Indeed, identification of risk factors for PTSD involves an analysis of the subjective (rather than objective) characteristics of the stress response. We also discuss research designs that may be useful in identifying risk factors for PTSD.

Table 1–1. DSM-IV diagnostic criteria for posttraumatic stress disorder

A. The person has been exposed to a traumatic event in which both of the following were present:

    (1) the person experienced, witnessed, or was confronted with an event or events that involved actual or threatened death or serious injury, or a threat to the physical integrity of self or others

    (2) the person's response involved intense fear, helplessness, or horror. **Note:** In children, this may be expressed instead by disorganized or agitated behavior

B. The traumatic event is persistently reexperienced in one (or more) of the following ways:

    (1) recurrent and intrusive distressing recollections of the event, including images, thoughts, or perceptions. **Note:** In young children, repetitive play may occur in which themes or aspects of the trauma are expressed.

    (2) recurrent distressing dreams of the event. **Note:** In children, there may be frightening dreams without recognizable content.

    (3) acting or feeling as if the traumatic event were recurring (includes a sense of reliving the experience, illusions, hallucinations, and dissociative flashback episodes, including those that occur on awakening or when intoxicated). **Note:** In young children, trauma-specific reenactment may occur.

    (4) intense psychological distress at exposure to internal or external cues that symbolize or resemble an aspect of the traumatic event

    (5) physiological reactivity on exposure to internal or external cues that symbolize or resemble an aspect of the traumatic event

C. Persistent avoidance of stimuli associated with the trauma and numbing of general responsiveness (not present before the trauma), as indicated by three (or more) of the following:

    (1) efforts to avoid thoughts, feelings, or conversations associated with the trauma

    (2) efforts to avoid activities, places, or people that arouse recollections of the trauma

    (3) inability to recall an important aspect of the trauma

    (4) markedly diminished interest or participation in significant activities

(continued)

Table 1–1. DSM-IV diagnostic criteria for posttraumatic stress disorder
(continued)

    (5) feeling of detachment or estrangement from others
    (6) restricted range of affect (e.g., unable to have loving feelings)
    (7) sense of a foreshortened future (e.g., does not expect to have a career, marriage, children, or a normal life span)

D. Persistent symptoms of increased arousal (not present before the trauma), as indicated by two (or more) of the following:

    (1) difficulty falling or staying asleep
    (2) irritability or outbursts of anger
    (3) difficulty concentrating
    (4) hypervigilance
    (5) exaggerated startle response

E. Duration of the disturbance (symptoms in Criteria B, C, and D) is more than 1 month.

F. The disturbance causes clinically significant distress or impairment in social, occupational, or other important areas of functioning.

Specify if:
    Acute: if duration of symptoms is less than 3 months
    Chronic: if duration of symptoms is 3 months or more
Specify if:
    With delayed onset: if onset of symptoms is at least 6 months after the stressor

Stress-Diathesis Models

The etiology of many psychiatric disorders has been studied in terms of the "stress-diathesis" model (Zubin and Spring 1977). In this conceptualization, exposure to a "stressor" (i.e., an event or agent to which an individual is exposed) is hypothesized to interact with preexisting personality characteristics and thereby to release or activate a "diathesis" (i.e., predisposition) toward a certain type of response to stress or illness in response to an environmental trigger. Neither the stressor nor the diathesis is viewed as necessary or sufficient to produce the condition. Implied in this model, however, is that both the stressor and the diathesis are necessary requirements for development of the illness.

Interestingly, in most psychiatric conditions, neither the stressor nor the diathesis has been specified clearly, and both have often proven very difficult to identify (Harvey et al. 1986). For example, in schizophrenia, no objective life events have been found to be correlated with the expression of schizophrenic symptoms despite the fact that genetic factors do not appear to fully account for the development of this disorder (Goldstein 1994). In depression, it has generally been thought that negative life events are associated with the onset of the disorder (Brown et al. 1986; Craig et al. 1987), but the potency of any particular stressor in eliciting a uniform depressive reaction in everyone exposed to such an event (or even everyone with the depressive diathesis, such as first-degree relatives of persons with depression) has not been adequately demonstrated. Moreover, the nature of the diatheses for schizophrenia and depression is only vaguely understood. Although several types of risk factors, particularly familial ones, have been hypothesized as important contributors to the development of these disorders, no consistent relationship between family history and depression has been observed. Indeed, the presence of both the diathesis and the stressor is typically inferred from the fact that neither on its own appears to be directly related to the psychiatric outcome (Gottesman and Shields 1982).

A stress-diathesis model is relatively easier to apply to PTSD compared with schizophrenia or depression because the definition of PTSD clearly specifies the type of stressor required. Only the presence of a diathesis need be inferred from the relatively limited incidence of PTSD following exposure to the stressors listed in criterion A of the DSM-IV criteria set. As a consequence, the study of the development of PTSD from a stress-diathesis perspective amounts in large part to careful study of the factors that predispose an individual to PTSD upon exposure to a sufficiently stressful event. However, because stressful events may vary in their ability to cause PTSD regardless of predisposition, and certain stressors may be more potent than others in terms of their ability to cause

PTSD, it is also essential to characterize stressor severity in a definite manner.

Characteristics of the Stressor

To critically evaluate the diatheses for PTSD, it is necessary first to establish how much of the variation in prevalence rates for chronic PTSD can legitimately be attributed to severity of the stressor. In the typical model of the relationship between stress and risk of chronic PTSD, referred to as the "linear" model, more intense stress exposure results in a higher risk of PTSD (Figure 1–1). This model has been the implicit backdrop for much of the research in combat-related PTSD, in which a positive correlation between intensity of combat exposure and risk rate for chronic PTSD has been

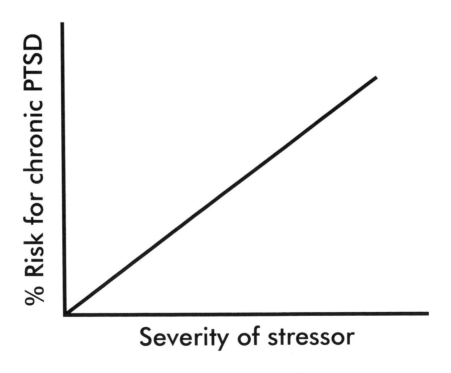

Figure 1–1.   Linear model of the relationship between stress and risk of developing chronic posttraumatic stress disorder (PTSD).

demonstrated (Foy et al. 1984), and is consistent with the classic dose-response relationship of the stressor and stress response described by Hans Selye (1936). This type of linear dose-response model does not consider the possibility of nonlinear relationships between stress and PTSD.

In contrast, an alternative model, based on empirical observations, has been proposed that takes into account nonlinear relationships (Figure 1–2). For example, concentration camp or prisoner-of-war (POW) experiences are traumatic events of such tremendous magnitude that nearly all exposed individuals report some PTSD symptoms (Goldstein et al. 1987; Yehuda et al. 1995b). Accordingly, there would be a high risk of developing chronic PTSD but little dose-response. Sexual assault is a potent trauma, and many victims report PTSD symptoms. In the case of sexual assault, the severity of the assault itself is associated with a further increase in risk for development of chronic PTSD (Resnick et al. 1992). In contrast, events such as motor vehicle accidents might be of a much

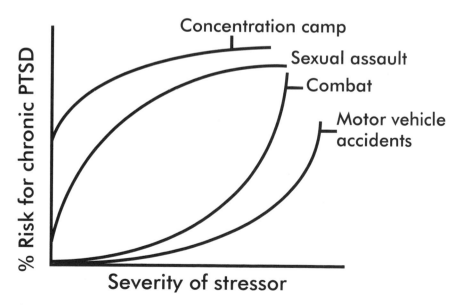

Figure 1–2.   Dose-response model of relationship between stress and risk of developing posttraumatic stress disorder (PTSD), taking into account nonlinear relationships.

lower potency, such that only in very severe instances of such events do PTSD symptoms develop (McFarlane et al. 1992, 1997). Thus, various traumatic stressors would be associated with marked variation in the general prevalence of chronic PTSD after exposure. This suggests that there might be qualitative differences in the consequences of exposure to different stressful situations.

In addition to assessing the type of traumatic event sustained, it is important to quantify the "dose," or severity, of the stressor objectively. Many attempts have been made to objectively quantify the intensity of traumatic events, and numerous scales now exist that attempt to measure specific aspects of particular events. For example, a rape exposure scale may include questions about the duration of the rape, type of penetrations, type (strangers, family members, acquaintances) and number of perpetrators, type of weapon(s) that was used, and whether physical injury was sustained. A combat exposure scale may include questions about frequency of being attacked by missiles, frequency and severity of physical injury, and experiences such as encountering dead bodies, witnessing the death of comrades, and witnessing or participating in atrocities.

Even if it were possible to accurately quantify the severity of the actual environmental events (assuming little or no retrospective reporting bias), it would still be necessary to assess the psychological state of victim at the time of the event (e.g., intoxication, fear) and immediately after the event in order to properly gauge the severity of the trauma. Such psychological assessment is required because the cognitive appraisal by the victim at the time of occurrence is an important mediator of the response to an event. Indeed, what actually happened may not have the same meaning to each individual exposed. Thus, the subjective impact of the event must be considered in assessing dose or severity. Some scales attempt to ask trauma victims to rate the intensity or impact of the event. However, ultimately, such rating can become confounded because often what is actually measured is the consequence of the stress response and not the severity of the event.

The foregoing discussion introduces a second difficulty in assessing stressor severity: the difficulty in knowing how much the assessment of trauma severity is influenced by the psychological response to the traumatic event. Indeed, there is some evidence that those with more severe symptoms are more likely retrospectively to score higher on measures of combat exposure as their symptoms grow worse, compared with at an earlier time point (Southwick et al. 1997). It may be that posttraumatic symptoms, by their nature, modify perceptions of the severity of the event (i.e., reexperiencing symptoms, including flashbacks, or other dissociative experiences, nightmares, intrusive thoughts, and psychogenic amnesia by definition imply some sense of memory distortion). Indeed, the severity and duration of symptoms may often confound assessments of the severity of events. Thus, the symptoms of PTSD, in and of themselves, may interfere with the recollection of both the objective and the subjective impact of the event, in addition to the retrospective biases that might occur as a function of time since the traumatic event.

Another issue that arises in attempting to quantify the effects of stress exposure is that of identification of the threshold needed for the development of PTSD. Insofar as there appear to be individual differences in the level of stress exposure required for the development of chronic PTSD, it is possible that the threshold for development of PTSD in a vulnerable individual is less than in other individuals and that relatively lower levels of stress could be associated with the development of PTSD (see Chapter 5, this volume). In this case, an "objective" measure of stress may not be particularly informative, because even a low level of stress exposure or response would still be associated with PTSD. In addition, in other, "invulnerable" individuals, the maximum measurable stress response may be less than the threshold for development of PTSD, a situation that could lead to a lack of correlation between biological response and risk for PTSD across individuals. Thus, what may be important is not how much stress one is exposed to or the specifics of the acute stress response, but rather individual differences in propensity for PTSD symptomatology to develop as a response to stress. Thus, consideration of predisposition to PTSD can unavoidably have an impact on measurement of the stress component of the diathesis-stress model.

Characteristics of a Diathesis

As defined in the previous subsection, a diathesis refers to a predisposing factor. These predisposing factors can be measured at a biological, cognitive, or behavioral level and may include the presence of personality traits or other psychiatric diagnoses. Diatheses can be inherited genetically, acquired in an intrauterine environment, or acquired postnatally through diet, toxic exposure, or other environmental experience (Harvey et al. 1986).

In the case of PTSD, proposed diatheses include gender and other demographic variables (see Chapter 2, this volume), prior trauma exposure (see Chapter 8), genetic (or at least familial) factors (see Chapters 3–5), neurocognitive factors (see Chapter 6), biological alterations (see Chapters 5 and 7), and personality characteristics (see Chapter 9). The experience of trauma, however, can affect at least some of these variables. Therefore, it is critical to discriminate between predisposing factors and consequences of stress. As will be more fully described later in this chapter, the best way to circumvent the problem of the effects of trauma on these variables is to assess these variables in individuals both before and after the traumatic event. These types of studies have not yet been performed for PTSD, but they will need to be done in order to confirm putative risk factors.

For a diathesis-stress model to be useful in the understanding of the development of PTSD, the predisposition must be definable and measurable before the onset of stress exposure. Only then could these measures be markers of vulnerability. For example, in schizophrenia research, levels of neurotransmitters, their by-products, and various related catabolic enzymes have been measured in "high risk" individuals in order to test biological hypotheses (Mednick and McNeil 1968). Various assessments of cognition and attention (Cornblatt and Keilp 1994), personality functioning assessments (Lenzenweger 1994), and measures of life events (Goldstein 1994) have also been used with these individuals to test cognitive, personality, and environmental exposure theories regarding the presence of risk-increasing factors. Applying this approach to PTSD research would involve consideration of whether any of the alterations associated with PTSD are indications of preexisting vulnerabilities rather than consequences of the traumatic event.

Acute Versus Chronic Stress Reactions

Traumatic situations, almost by definition, cause some level of emotional upset in individuals exposed to them. Indeed, it has been well documented that in the immediate aftermath of trauma, most exposed individuals do report some type of emotional changes (Foa 1997; Koopman et al. 1994). Importantly, however, the majority of individuals who are negatively affected in the immediate aftermath of a traumatic event will show substantial improvement in stress symptoms within a few months or years (Foa et al. 1991; McFarlane 1992). In this sense, one dimension of predisposition to PTSD may be an inability to recover and readjust soon after exposure to trauma. It is conceivable, for instance, that certain stressors cause acute stress reactions in the majority of exposed individuals without necessarily leading to chronic PTSD. Thus, it is important for researchers to separate the acute effects of stress from the development of PTSD (see Chapter 8, this volume).

Ultimately, distinguishing between the acute and chronic effects of a traumatic event requires a longitudinal approach in which individuals are evaluated immediately after trauma exposure and then reevaluated at some later point. Very little such research has been done in PTSD. As described below, stressors may vary in their potency, and even within stressors dose-response effects may be important as well. However, only a subset of individuals may be vulnerable to the development of chronic PTSD, regardless of the type and severity of trauma.

Discrimination of Correlates of PTSD From Effects of Specific Stressors

Methodological Issues

PTSD has been associated with a broad array of biological and cognitive abnormalities. As alluded to earlier in this chapter, comparisons between trauma survivors with PTSD and nonexposed control subjects do not allow a determination of whether abnormalities 1) are consequences of chronic PTSD, 2) are consequences of stress exposure, or 3) reflect vulnerability to the disorder. However, inclusion of a group of trauma-exposed subjects without PTSD greatly enhances the information that can be obtained from cross-sectional studies. If any abnormality is uniformly present in individuals with PTSD but absent in stress-exposed individuals without PTSD, then the abnormality must be a consequence of either the PTSD or a predisposing factor, but it is not a direct consequence of exposure to the traumatic event.

Differences within individuals with PTSD on any of these variables may provide information about the effects of specific stressors. Characteristics of trauma survivors without PTSD may clarify further issues regarding possible "invulnerability" factors. Finally, comparisons of individuals who vary in their level of exposure to the same stressor may provide information about the effects of different "doses" of stress exposure. Thus, learning about risk factors for PTSD must involve systematically ruling out the variables that are present in trauma survivors without PTSD.

Specificity of Stress Effects on Neuroendocrine Indices in Trauma Survivors

As an illustration of the methodological issues raised above, we present neuroendocrine data from male Holocaust survivors and Vietnam War veterans. Some of these data have been published elsewhere (Yehuda et al. 1995a). Subjects were asked to collect a 24-hour urine specimen, which was stored frozen until it was assayed for the determination of cortisol, catecholamines, and catecholamine metabolites (for detailed descriptions of the methods used to assay these neurochemicals, see Yehuda et al. 1990, 1992).

Measures of urinary cortisol and monoamine levels for six groups of men are graphically depicted in Figure 1–3. The six groups represented are 1) Holocaust survivors with PTSD ($n = 13$), Holocaust survivors without PTSD ($n = 10$), and men of comparable age who had not been exposed to trauma ($n = 13$); and 2) Vietnam combat veterans with PTSD ($n = 19$), Vietnam combat veterans without PTSD ($n = 15$), and men of comparable age who had not been exposed to trauma ($n = 25$).

As can be seen in Figure 1–3, individuals with PTSD had significantly lower cortisol levels than the trauma-exposed and non–trauma exposed groups in both subject populations. In both subject populations, mean urinary cortisol excretion in trauma-exposed subjects without PTSD did not differ from that in nonexposed comparison subjects. In contrast, catecholamine levels tended to be directionally different in Holocaust survivors and Vietnam veterans with PTSD. Holocaust survivors with PTSD showed significantly lower norepinephrine levels compared with Holocaust survivors without PTSD and non–trauma exposed subjects, whereas Vietnam veterans showed a significantly higher mean norepinephrine excretion compared with combat veterans without PTSD and age-comparable nonexposed subjects.

These data suggest that PTSD may have a specific biological "signature" in terms of cortisol level. However, other biological indices, although found to be significantly different from those in appropriate comparison subjects, may actually vary in different groups with PTSD. These results show that biological alterations that are specifically related to PTSD can potentially be discriminated from effects of stress exposure. Furthermore, these data suggest that it will be necessary to identify the similarities and differences in the consequences of exposure to different types of traumatic stressors and/or trauma survivors. Indeed, Holocaust survivors and combat veterans differ not only in the type of trauma sustained but also in other important variables such as their age at assessment, their age at traumatization, duration of symptoms, presence of comorbid psychopathology and/or substance abuse, and variables such as education and cultural differences. Therefore, it is not clear whether the norepinephrine levels observed reflect any of these differences, or even if they reflect some other individual characteristics of the subjects. However, it is clear that norepinephrine levels probably cannot be used as a marker for PTSD across all subject groups, and therefore it is unlikely that this neurochemical is a risk factor.

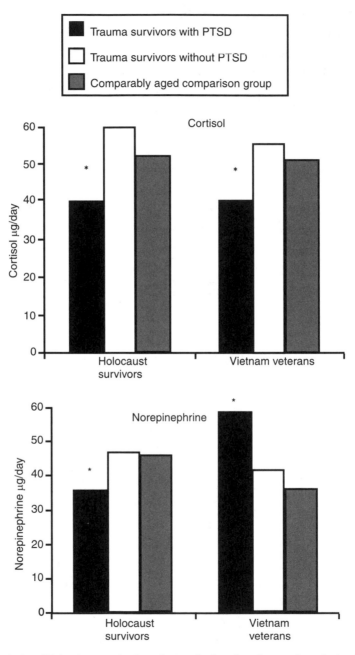

Figure 1–3. Urinary cortisol and catecholamine (norepinephrine) excretion in trauma survivors with and without posttraumatic stress disorder (PTSD) and comparably aged control subjects.

Factors Accounting for Interindividual Differences in Risk for PTSD

As noted above, the risk for development of PTSD after exposure to trauma is less than 100%. Since the trauma exposure alone fails to account for the development of the disorder, individual differences must be responsible for the variations in risk. Differences associated with predisposing factors must therefore be responsible for differential risk for PTSD across different individuals. These individual differences include previous trauma exposure, developmental experiences (see Chapter 2, this volume), differences in personality characteristics (see Chapter 9), differences in psychophysiological reactivity (see Chapter 7), neurocognitive and intellectual factors (see Chapter 6), history of previous psychopathology (see Chapter 2), and basic individual differences such as gender (see Chapter 2). As explored in other chapters in this volume, many of these aspects of individual differences have been found to correlate with variations in risk for the development of PTSD after exposure to trauma.

Research Designs for Identification of Putative Risk Factors

Clearly, the ideal way to study the development of a posttraumatic reaction is to examine individuals before and after exposure to the traumatic stressor. With this approach, there is no logical possibility that the trauma exposure influenced the overall results. Similarly, there is no possibility that the consequences of chronic PTSD and of its treatment (e.g., social avoidance, substance abuse, pharmacological treatment) could influence the assessment data collected.

However, this design is not generally feasible. First, the rate of trauma exposure is low in the general population. Second, not all individuals exposed to trauma develop PTSD—that is the point of this volume. Several other research methods can provide initial (pretrauma) data to aid in the hypothesis generation procedure for identifying risk factors. These designs include archival (retrospective), epidemiological, family, genetic, and longitudinal studies.

Archival (Retrospective) Studies

Studies of archival information are often referred to as "follow-back" studies. In this design, record information on individuals is obtained from data collected prior to trauma exposure. These records can be obtained from school records, military service records, occupational testing files, and formal mental health treatment records (such as those in the Scandinavian countries where mental health registers are kept). The principal benefit of such studies is that of uncontaminated records that were collected without any knowledge of the subsequent trauma exposure.

Archival information includes information from records of medical health, pregnancy and birth complications, academic achievement, intellectual functioning, and treatment for psychiatric conditions. Information on behavioral disorders, including that contained in detention records, military misconduct records, and formal psychiatric assessments, can also be examined. Finally, military service records, including information on combat exposure, military decorations (for valor or purple hearts), and location of service, can be used to identify groups of individuals who have relatively similar stress exposure histories.

The archival design is probably best used for hypothesis generation. A major limitation of this method is bias in the data collected. Only the information contained in an archive can be examined, and these records have often proven to be incomplete or nonspecific. Finally, use of mental health records is another possible source of bias because of the low rate of service utilization of many PTSD populations prior to the trauma. Similarly, diagnostic information collected from clinical files is notably unreliable compared with research diagnoses on the same cases. At the same time, recall bias, including effects of the trauma itself on recollections of the event, is avoided.

Cross-Sectional Epidemiological Studies

Cross-sectional epidemiological studies focus on the occurrence of PTSD in circumscribed populations. As described in the next chapter, there is often useful information to be obtained through examination of the covariates of PTSD. For example, correlations between age, gender, and other aspects of psychopathology and PTSD can be examined in detail. The rates of PTSD after a generalized trauma (e.g., earthquake, wildfire, hurricane) can also be determined from these studies. Although these studies are cross-sectional and not developmental, much can be learned about risk factors from identification of correlates (and noncorrelates) of any illness or condition.

Family Studies

Many psychiatric and nonpsychiatric illnesses run in families. Although, usually, a determination that a disorder is familial suggests a genetic component to an illness, there are other possible explanations for nongenetic familial associations. For instance, Huntington's disease and mental retardation associated with lead poisoning are both highly familial diseases. However, the latter illness is entirely the result of biological environmental factors, and the former is transmitted by a single dominant gene with no contribution from the environment.

As described elsewhere in this volume (see Chapter 4), studies of family members of individuals with PTSD can answer a number of questions about risk factors for this condition. One of the major advantages of a family study is that information regarding any of the domains of potential risk factors can be addressed.

Genetic Studies

While not all familial conditions are genetically transmitted, all genetic conditions are familial. Thus, a genetic study, typically involving studies of concordance for the disorder or putative risk factors between monozygotic and dizygotic twins, involves a special case of the family study (see Chapter 3, this volume). Specifically, examination of the concordance of putative risk factors across monozygotic as compared with dizygotic co-twins can provide information about the genetic status of the risk factor. Similarly, concordance of PTSD across similarly stress-exposed twins can answer broader questions about the genetic status of PTSD.

Longitudinal Studies

PTSD is in many ways an ideal disorder to study with a longitudinal design, because this disorder, by definition, occurs after trauma exposure. Thus, risk factors should be present and identifiable before the traumatic stressor, with PTSD occurring only after the trauma in some individuals. The ideal research design would involve identifying high- and low-risk groups, based on some combinations of the predispositions just described for the development of PTSD, and observing the longitudinal course of the reactions of these individuals to traumatic events. It is at least theoretically possible to perform a prospective study of individuals at high risk for the development of PTSD if high-risk groups can be identified on the basis of theoretically high risk of PTSD after trauma exposure and/or high risk of exposure to traumatic events.

That said, there are some basic limitations of such a research design. First, as noted above, because there is considerable variation in PTSD risk associated with trauma exposure, and because this risk varies across type of exposure, such a design is logistically complicated, not to mention expensive. It is not clear, for example, who should be followed and for how long. It is also not clear how one goes about selecting subjects who have a relatively high probability of developing PTSD.

In considering groups of individuals at risk for PTSD, there are two strategies. The first is to select subjects on the basis of their increased risk for experiencing a traumatic event due to occupational hazards (e.g., firefighting personnel, police, EMS [emergency medical service] workers) or other planned exposures (e.g., military recruits who will be deployed to war zones). The second is to follow up individuals based on their increased risk for developing PTSD due to familial PTSD (e.g., see Chapters 3–5, this volume). A combination of these strategies would entail following up individuals with familial risk factors that are further augmented by risk from environmental events (e.g., sons of fathers with combat experience who themselves will be deployed to war zones, adult children of firefighting personnel, police, or EMS workers who themselves enter these professions).

Repeated Trauma

One finding that has emerged consistently from longitudinal research on PTSD is that previous trauma exposure is a risk factor for development of PTSD upon subsequent exposure to a new event. One use of this finding in a study designed to identify individuals at high risk of developing PTSD is to examine trauma survivors without evidence of PTSD and follow them longitudinally until the experience of the next trauma. Differences between individuals after the first trauma could then be used to predict those who will develop PTSD at subsequent trauma exposure. This design would be particularly powerful for study of groups in situations where a new possible trauma is likely to be experienced in the immediate future, such as firefighting personnel, EMS workers, and ER (emergency room) staff. Given the high frequency of trauma exposure in these groups, information regarding predictors of increased risk of PTSD after subsequent traumas could be available within a very brief period.

Multiple Risk Factors

A recent study examining Israeli combat veterans found that those whose parents were Holocaust survivors were more likely to manifest PTSD symptoms after combat exposure than those whose parents had not been directly exposed to the Holocaust (Solomon et al. 1988). Family history of PTSD, or at least multiple trauma, was shown to interact with subsequent trauma exposure.

Thus, family history of PTSD, including among siblings, could be studied in environmentally high-risk populations in order to identify individuals at especially high risk. This longitudinal design could also be particularly useful in the study of "high risk" individuals who are expected to experience high rates of trauma.

Conclusion

PTSD is not simply a result of exposure to trauma. There is variation in the ability of stressors to cause PTSD and in the vulnerability of individuals to the development of PTSD regardless of the stressor. Thus, adoption of a stress-diathesis model appears to be the only logical way to approach the study of the development of this disorder. Considerable information can be gained even from cross-sectional studies if clear conceptualizations of the differences between predisposing factors and stress exposure can be developed. Longitudinal designs provide a powerful methodology to study development of PTSD. These studies avoid many of the problems of archival (retrospective) and cross-sectional epidemiological designs and allow for clear separation of potential risk factors for trauma from the consequences of the experience. Although several pragmatic issues require consideration, PTSD is in many ways an ideal disorder for investigations with strategies identified to differentiate aspects of stress exposure and predisposing factors associated with individual differences. As the later chapters in this book indicate, this research has already made considerable progress.

References

American Psychiatric Association: Diagnostic and Statistical Manual of Mental Disorders, 4th Edition. Washington, DC, American Psychiatric Association, 1994

Breslau N, Davis GC, Andreski P, et al: Traumatic events and posttraumatic stress disorder in an urban population of young adults. Arch Gen Psychiatry 48:216–222, 1991

Brown GW, Bifulco A, Harris T, et al: Life stress, chronic subclinical symptoms and vulnerability to clinical depression. J Affect Disord 11: 1–19, 1986

Cornblatt BA, Keilp JG: Impaired attention, genetics, and pathophysiology of schizophrenia. Schizophr Bull 20:31–46, 1994

Craig TKJ, Brown GW, Harris TO: Depression in the general population: comparability of survey results. Br J Psychiatry 150:707–708, 1987

Davidson JRT, Hughes D, Blazer D, et al: Posttraumatic stress disorder in the community: an epidemiological study. Psychol Med 21:1–9, 1991

Foa EB: Psychological processes related to recovery from a trauma and an effective treatment for PTSD. Ann N Y Acad Sci 821:410–424, 1997

Foa EB, Rothbaum BO, Riggs DS, et al: Treatment of posttraumatic stress disorder in rape victims: a comparison between cognitive-behavioral procedures and counseling. J Consult Clin Psychol 59:715–723, 1991

Foy DW, Sipprelle RC, Rueger DB, et al: Etiology of posttraumatic stress disorder in Vietnam veterans. J Consult Clin Psychol 40:1323–1328, 1984

Goldstein G, Van Kammen W, Shelly C, et al: Survivors of imprisonment in the Pacific theatre during World War II. Am J Psychiatry 144:1210–1213, 1987

Goldstein MJ: Family expressed emotion, childhood-onset depression, and childhood-onset schizophrenia spectrum disorders: is expressed emotion a nonspecific correlate of child psychopathology or a specific risk factor for depression? J Abnorm Child Psychol 22:129–146, 1994

Gottesman II, Shields J: Schizophrenia: The Epigenetic Puzzle. New York, Oxford University Press, 1982

Harvey PD, Walker E, Wielgus MS: Psychological markers of vulnerability to schizophrenia: research and future directions. Progress in Experimental Personality Research 14:231–267, 1986

Helzer JE, Robins LN, McEvoy L: Posttraumatic stress disorder in the general population. N Engl J Med 317:1630–1634, 1987

Koopman C, Classen C, Spiegel D: Predictors of posttraumatic stress symptoms among survivors of the Oakland/Berkeley, CA, firestorm. Am J Psychiatry 151:888–894, 1994

Lenzenweger MF: Psychometric high-risk paradigm, perceptual aberrations, and schizotypy: an update. Schizophr Bulll 20:121–135, 1994

McFarlane AC: Multiple diagnoses in posttraumatic stress disorder in the victims of a natural disaster. J Nerv Ment Dis 180:498–504, 1992

McFarlane AC, Atchison M, Yehuda R: The acute stress response following motor vehicle accidents and its relation to PTSD. Ann N Y Acad Sci 821:437–441, 1997

Mednick S, McNeil T: Current methodology on research on the etiology of schizophrenia: serious difficulties that suggest the use of the high-risk group method. Psychol Bull 70:681–693, 1968

Resnick HS, Kilpatrick DG, Best CL, et al: Vulnerability-stress factors in development of posttraumatic stress disorder. J Nerv Ment Dis 180: 424–430, 1992

Rothbaum BO, Foa EB, Riggs DS, et al: A prospective examination of posttraumatic stress disorder in rape victims. J Trauma Stress 5:455–475, 1992

Solomon Z, Kotler M, Mikulincer M: Combat-related posttraumatic stress disorder among second-generation Holocaust survivors: preliminary findings. Am J Psychiatry 145:865–868, 1988

Southwick SM, Morgan CA, Nicolau A, et al: Consistency of memory for combat-related traumatic events in veterans of Desert Storm. Am J Psychiatry 154:173–177, 1997

Yehuda R, McFarlane AC: Conflict between current knowledge about posttraumatic stress disorder and its original conceptual basis. Am J Psychiatry 152:1705–1713, 1995

Yehuda R, Southwick SM, Nussbaum G, et al: Low urinary cortisol excretion in patients with posttraumatic stress disorder. J Nerv Ment Dis 178:366–369, 1990

Yehuda R, Southwick SM, Ma X, et al: Urinary catecholamine excretion and severity of symptoms in PTSD. J Nerv Ment Dis 180:321–325, 1992

Yehuda R, Kahana BK, Binder-Brynes K, et al: Low urinary cortisol in Holocaust survivors with posttraumatic stress disorder. Am J Psychiatry 152:982–986, 1995a

Yehuda R, Kahana B, Schmeidler J, et al: The impact of cumulative life-time trauma and recent stress on current posttraumatic stress disorder symptoms in Holocaust survivors. Am J Psychiatry 152:1815–1818, 1995b

Zubin JS, Spring B: Vulnerability: a new view of schizophrenia. J Abnorm Psychol 86:103–126, 1977

Chapter 2

Epidemiological Risk Factors for Trauma and PTSD

Ronald C. Kessler, Ph.D., Amanda Sonnega, Ph.D.,
Evelyn Bromet, Ph.D., Michael Hughes, Ph.D.,
Christopher B. Nelson, Ph.D., M.P.H., and
Naomi Breslau, Ph.D.

Although it has long been known that pathological stress response syndromes can result from exposure to war (Freud 1919/1955), sexual assault (Burgess and Holstrum 1974), and other types of trauma (Grinker and Spiegel 1945; Horowitz 1976; Lindemann 1944; Parad et al. 1976), the codification of diagnostic criteria

---

Some of the material reported here appeared in a previous article by the authors (Kessler et al. 1995).

The National Comorbidity Survey (NCS) is a collaborative epidemiological investigation of the prevalences, causes, and consequences of psychiatric morbidity and comorbidity in the United States. This survey was supported by the National Institute of Mental Health (RO1 MH46376, RO1 MH52861), with supplemental support from the National Institute on Drug Abuse (through a supplement to MH46376) and the W. T. Grant Foundation (90135190), Ronald C. Kessler, Principal Investigator. Preparation for this report was also supported by a Research Scientist Award to Dr. Kessler (K05 MH00507). Collaborating NCS sites and investigators are as follows: The Addiction Research Foundation (Robin Room), Duke University Medical Center (Dan Blazer, Marvin Swartz), Harvard Medical School (Richard Frank, Ronald Kessler), Johns Hopkins University (James Anthony, William Eaton, Philip Leaf), Max Planck Institute of Psychiatry Clinical Institute (Hans-Ulrich Wittchen), Medical College of Virginia (Kenneth Kendler), University of Miami (R. Jay Turner), University of Michigan (Lloyd Johnston, Roderick Little), New York University (Patrick Shrout), SUNY—Stony Brook (Evelyn Bromet), and Washington University School of Medicine (Linda Cottler, Andrew Heath). A complete list of all NCS publications, along with abstracts, study documentation, interview schedules, and the raw NCS public use data files, can be obtained directly from the NCS Home page by using the URL: http://www.umich.edu/ncsum/.

for these responses in DSM-III (American Psychiatric Association 1980) under the diagnosis of posttraumatic stress disorder (PTSD) stimulated a considerable amount of new research. Most of this work has focused on victims of specific traumas such as criminal victimization (Kilpatrick and Resnick 1992; Kilpatrick et al. 1987), sexual assault (Frank and Anderson 1987; Pynoos and Nader 1988), exposure to natural disaster (Goenjian et al. 1994; Koopman et al. 1994), and combat exposure (Kulka et al. 1990; Solomon et al. 1994). The empirical information and conceptual refinements generated by this research have advanced our understanding of traumatic stress responses and have led to revisions of the diagnostic criteria for PTSD in DSM-III-R (American Psychiatric Association 1987) and DSM-IV (American Psychiatric Association 1994).

However, despite this growing body of work on the extent to which PTSD is associated with specific traumas, limited epidemiological data are available on the total population prevalence of PTSD, the kinds of traumatic events most likely to cause PTSD, and the epidemiological risk factors for PTSD. In this chapter, we present data on these issues from the National Comorbidity Survey (NCS) (Kessler et al. 1994, 1995). We also briefly report preliminary results from an even more recent local survey and discuss important conceptual and methodological considerations for future research.

Previous Epidemiological Research on PTSD

The two earliest general population prevalence studies of PTSD using DSM-III criteria, carried out as part of the Epidemiologic Catchment Area (ECA) program in St. Louis (Helzer et al. 1987) and North Carolina (Davidson et al. 1991), reported that PTSD is a rare disorder, with lifetime prevalence of only about 1%. A lifetime prevalence of 2.6% was subsequently found in the control sample of a case-control study of persons exposed to the Mount St. Helens volcanic eruption that used the same measurement methodology as the ECA study (Shore et al. 1989). However, subsequent studies using DSM-III-R criteria reported much higher rates. In a national telephone survey of women, Resnick and colleagues (1993) found that 12.3% of respondents (17.9% of those exposed to a traumatic event) had a lifetime history of DSM-III-R PTSD. Breslau and colleagues (1991) administered the revised version of the Diagnostic Interview Schedule for DSM-III-R to a sample of young adults enrolled in an HMO in Detroit and found that 11.3% of the women (30.7% of those exposed to a traumatic event) and 6.0% of the men (14.0% of those exposed) had a lifetime history of PTSD.

Several factors might be involved in the much higher prevalences of PTSD found in the DSM-III-R studies compared with the DSM-III studies, including differences in diagnostic criteria, assessment procedures, and sample characteristics (Croyle and Loftus 1992; Koss 1983). Resnick and colleagues (1993) noted that the anonymity of telephone interviews may have contributed to the fact that so many women in their study reported traumatic experiences. Breslau and colleagues (1991) noted that recall bias was minimized in their study because of the young age of the respondents in their sample, a factor that possibly explains why their prevalence estimate was comparatively high. An additional factor of considerable importance is that the assessment of PTSD in the ECA and Mount St. Helen's studies used a very complex diagnostic stem question that was cognitively challenging in that it required respondents to pay close attention to the question and to do a good deal of memory work. The question format was also potentially quite embarrassing in that it required the respondent to say out loud what happened. A rape victim, for example, had to say "I was raped." These problems were reduced in the Resnick and Breslau studies. As will be described later in this chapter, subsequent methodological studies carried out in preparation for the NCS documented that data collection problems such as those in the early studies lead to underestimation of PTSD.

Only limited information is available on the types of traumatic experiences most likely to cause PTSD. Many of the traumas identified as likely to cause PTSD are quite common (Breslau et al. 1991; Resnick et al. 1993), so the stipulation in the DSM system that the trauma must be outside the range of usual human experience is difficult to defend (Solomon and Canino 1990). Yet ignoring this stipulation and allowing people with intrusive recollections of any stressful event to be evaluated as potential "cases" could dilute the meaning of PTSD as a stress-response syndrome (March 1992). One unresolved issue in this debate concerns the risk of PTSD after trauma exposure. The DSM system implicitly assumes that risk of PTSD will be uniformly high among those exposed to traumatic events. Yet a review of trauma studies shows that, on average, only about one-fourth of trauma victims develop PTSD (Green 1994). We extend this investigation in what follows by examining the extent to which risk of PTSD varies across types of trauma.

The relationships between a variety of demographic predictors and PTSD must be taken into account. In what follows, we study the relationships of these variables with both trauma exposure and conditional risk of PTSD after exposure. A number of these significant predictors of PTSD are found to predict trauma exposure but not conditional risk of PTSD after exposure. A more common pattern is for the predictors to be unrelated to trauma exposure but significantly related to conditional risk of PTSD. The strongest predictors, however, are related both to trauma exposure and to conditional risk.

Another important consideration in understanding PTSD is the high rate of comorbidity. Kulka and colleagues (1990) reported that more than 90% of the combat veterans with a history of PTSD in the National Vietnam Veterans Readjustment Study had a history of some other DSM-III-R disorder as assessed with the Diagnostic Interview Schedule. Helzer and colleagues (1987) and Breslau and co-workers (1991) reported that nearly 80% of respondents with PTSD had experienced other psychiatric disorders. Rates of comorbidity between 62% (Davidson et al. 1991) and 92% (Shore et al. 1989) have been reported in other population-based surveys of PTSD. Research in both treatment samples (Davidson et al. 1990; Mellman et al. 1992) and population-based samples (Resnick et al. 1991) has used information on age at onset to show that prior history of other psychiatric disorders is associated with increased risk of subsequent PTSD. An expanded analysis of these effects is presented in this chapter.

The National Comorbidity Survey

The NCS was designed to study the distribution, correlates, and consequences of psychiatric disorders in the United States. The survey was based on a stratified, multistage area probability sample of persons ranging in age from 15 to 54 years in the noninstitutionalized civilian population in the 48 coterminous states. This sample included a supplemental sample of students living in campus group housing, selected from a widely dispersed sampling range. A special nonresponse survey was carried out to ascertain and then statistically adjust for nonresponse bias. Interviews were administered face to face in the homes of respondents from the fall of 1990 through the winter of 1992. The response rate was 82.4%. A total of 8,098 respondents participated in the survey. Further details about the sampling methodology of the NCS have been reported elsewhere (Kessler et al. 1994, 1995).

The NCS interview was administered in two parts, each of which took somewhat more than 1 hour to complete. Part I included the core diagnostic interview, a brief risk factor battery, and an inventory of sociodemographic information. Part II included a much more detailed risk factor battery and consideration of secondary diagnoses, including PTSD, that were not included in the core diagnostic interview. Part I was administered to all 8,098 respondents. Budgetary constraints required that we administer Part II to only a subsample of respondents, comprising those ages 15 to 24 years (99.4% of whom completed Part II), all others who screened positive for any lifetime diagnosis in Part I (98.1% of whom completed Part II), and a random subsample of other respondents (99.0% of whom completed Part II). A total of 5,877 respondents completed Part II.

The main diagnostic interview in the NCS was a modified version of the Composite International Diagnostic Interview (CIDI; World Health Organization 1990a), a fully structured interview developed by the World Health Organization to foster cross-cultural epidemiological research by producing diagnoses according to the definitions and criteria of both DSM-III-R and the Diagnostic Criteria for Research of ICD-10 (Robins et al. 1988). Diagnoses were generated by the use of the CIDI diagnostic program (World Health Organization 1990b). In the NCS, we used the diagnostic section for antisocial personality disorder from the Diagnostic Interview Schedule. To assess PTSD, we used a modified version of the Revised Diagnostic Interview Schedule (Breslau et al. 1991) in order to be consistent with the assessment in recent United States epidemiological surveys of PTSD (Breslau et al. 1991; Resnick et al. 1993). In addition to the Revised Diagnostic Interview Schedule symptom questions, additional questions were asked about how quickly the symptoms began after the trauma, how long the symptoms continued for "at least a few times a week," and how recently the respondent had any symptom associated with the trauma.

We made three important modifications to the Revised Diagnostic Interview Schedule PTSD section based on preliminary methodological studies. The first involved the method for inquiring about traumatic stressors. Unlike the Revised Diagnostic Interview Schedule, which contains a single stem question about the lifetime history of traumatic events directly experienced by oneself, with a list of such events provided, and a second question about exposure to traumas experienced by others, the NCS attempted to focus memory search by asking separate questions about each of 12 types of trauma. Pilot studies for the NCS showed that this approach leads to much more focused memory search and more complete reporting of traumatic experiences than can be obtained with the original Diagnostic Interview Schedule questions. This result is consistent with the results from other methodological studies documenting improved reporting accuracy of several different types of life experiences when recall is aided with concrete lists rather than more global open-ended questions (Kessler and Wethington 1991; Martin et al. 1986). The first 11 questions in this series were about events and experiences that qualify as traumas in DSM-III-R (Table 2–1). Question 12 was an open-ended question about "any other terrible experience that most people never go through." Open-ended responses to this question were subsequently coded as either qualifying under DSM-III-R criterion A (e.g., discovering a dead body) or not qualifying (e.g., normal bereavement). Responses that did not refer to specific events, were vague, or were

Table 2–1. National Comorbidity Survey items about events and experiences qualifying as DSM-III-R–defined traumas

Did any of these events ever happen to you?

1. You had direct combat experience in a war.
2. You were involved in a life-threatening accident.
3. You were involved in a fire, flood, or natural disaster.
4. You witnessed someone being badly injured or killed.
5. You were raped (someone had sexual intercourse with you when you did not want to by threatening you or using some degree of force).
6. You were sexually molested (someone touched or felt your genitals when you did not want them to).
7. You were seriously physically attacked or assaulted.
8. You were physically abused as a child.
9. You were seriously neglected as a child.
10. You were threatened with a weapon, held captive, or kidnapped.
11. You suffered a great shock because one of the events on this list happened to someone close to you.
12. Other ("any other terrible experience that most people never go through").

confounded with PTSD (e.g., biological depression) were eliminated from consideration.

The second modification involved presenting the 12 traumatic experiences to respondents in the form of a booklet. The rationale for taking this approach was based on evidence from pilot studies that respondents are sometimes reluctant to admit the occurrence of embarrassing and stigmatizing traumas such as rape and sexual abuse. Interviewers asked about these experiences by number (e.g., "Did you ever experience event number one on the list?" "How old were you when event number one first happened?") rather than by name. In the ECA, in comparison, the respondent was asked whether he or she had ever had any trauma and, if so, to describe the trauma. Our methodological studies showed, not surprisingly, that many respondents were very reluctant to do this, especially when the traumas were potentially embarrassing. Respondents were much more likely to say yes to the question "Did event number five ever occur to you?" in conjunction with a written list in which "rape" is event number five than to volunteer "Yes, I was raped" in response to an open-ended question.

The third modification, which also represents a limitation of the NCS, involved evaluating PTSD symptoms for only one event per respondent. In the Revised Diagnostic Interview Schedule, these symptoms are evaluated for up to three events. In the NCS, the limitation of one event per respondent was imposed because of time and budget constraints. As a result, we were able to determine whether each respondent developed PTSD after the one lifetime traumatic experience that he or she nominated as "most upsetting," but we had no way of knowing whether the respondent developed PTSD after one of his or her other lifetime traumas. Therefore, our estimates of lifetime prevalence are lower bound estimates. As will be described later in this chapter, however, we subsequently developed an expanded evaluation of DSM-IV PTSD for the revised CIDI 2.1 (World Health Organization 1997) that solves this problem. This new interview also adds an extremely important refinement, in which PTSD is evaluated not only for the self-defined "most upsetting" trauma but also for "random" traumas.

A small validation survey of the NCS PTSD module was conducted with a probability sample of 29 NCS respondents who had reported the occurrence of a lifetime trauma in the NCS. These individuals were reinterviewed by trained clinical interviewers with a modified version of the PTSD module from SCALUP, an instrument that includes items from both the Structured Clinical Interview for DSM-III-R—Patient Version (SCID-P) (Spitzer et al. 1989) and the Schedule for Affective Disorders and Schizophrenia—Lifetime Version (SADS-L) (Endicott and Spitzer 1978). SCALUP was developed by researchers at the Harvard-Brown Anxiety Disorders Research Program (Keller et al. 1987; Warshaw et al. 1993). Respondents who received a diagnosis ($n = 18$) were oversampled compared with those who did not receive a diagnosis ($n = 11$). Interviewers were blind to the NCS diagnoses. A weighted analysis that took this oversampling into consideration led to an estimated kappa (standard error) of 0.75 (0.11). Positive predictive value was 1.0, and negative predictive value was 0.88 (.08), values which suggest that the assessment of PTSD used in the NCS somewhat underestimates the prevalence that would have been obtained if clinical interviewers had administered SCALUP to the entire sample. The NCS estimated that the lifetime prevalence of PTSD in the total sample was 7.8% (Kessler et al. 1995).

Prevalence of Trauma

Estimates of the prevalence of the traumatic experiences that lead to PTSD were analyzed based on sex of respondent (first set of columns in Table 2–2). In the NCS sample, 60.7% of men and 51.2% of women reported having experienced at least one traumatic event. Consistent with previous research (Kilpatrick and Resnick 1992), the majority of respondents with a lifetime trauma actually experienced two or more traumas. The most prevalent traumas were witnessing someone being badly injured or killed; being involved in a fire, flood, or natural disaster; and being involved in a life-threatening accident. Men were significantly more likely than women to report each of these three as well as physical attacks, combat experience, being threatened with a weapon, being held captive, or being kidnapped. Women were significantly more likely than men to report rape, sexual molestation, childhood parental neglect, and childhood physical abuse.

Differential Risk of PTSD Across Trauma Types

Consistent with previous research reviewed by March (1992) and Kilpatrick and Resnick (1992), the risk of PTSD among respondents who had experienced trauma was found to vary significantly by type of trauma (second set of columns in Table 2–2). The traumas most often related to PTSD among both men and women were rape, childhood physical abuse, and childhood neglect. All three of these traumas were significantly more likely to be experienced by women than by men. Thus, although men were more likely than women to experience at least one trauma overall, women were

Table 2–2. Lifetime prevalence of trauma and risk of posttraumatic stress disorder (PTSD) associated with each trauma in the National Comorbidity Survey

Trauma	Lifetime prevalence of trauma		Lifetime prevalence of PTSD among respondents exposed to each trauma[a]		Lifetime prevalence of PTSD associated with each trauma[b]	
	Men	Women	Men	Women	Men	Women
	% (SE)	% (SE)	% (SE)	% (SE)	% (SE)	% (SE)
Rape	0.7* (0.2)	9.2 (0.8)	46.4 (13.6)	48.0 (5.1)	65.0 (15.6)	45.9 (5.9)
Molestation	2.8* (0.5)	12.3 (1.0)	24.8 (7.4)	33.2 (4.0)	12.2* (5.3)	26.5 (4.0)
Physical attack	11.1* (1.0)	6.9 (0.9)	15.3* (2.7)	39.1 (5.5)	1.8* (0.9)	21.3 (7.3)
Combat	6.4* (0.9)	0.0 (…)	29.2* (6.3)	…	38.8* (9.9)	…
Shock	11.4 (1.1)	12.4 (1.1)	14.9* (2.4)	26.2 (2.9)	4.4* (1.4)	10.4 (2.0)
Threat w/weapon	19.0* (1.3)	6.8 (0.6)	11.6* (1.8)	40.8 (4.4)	1.9* (0.8)	32.6 (7.8)
Accident	25.0* (1.2)	13.8 (1.1)	12.3* (2.0)	23.8 (3.4)	6.3 (1.8)	8.8 (4.3)
Natural disaster w/fire	18.9* (1.4)	15.2 (1.2)	10.4* (1.9)	17.4 (2.3)	3.7 (1.8)	5.4 (3.8)
Witness	35.6* (2.0)	14.5 (0.7)	9.8* (1.3)	20.1 (2.5)	6.4 (1.2)	7.5 (1.7)
Childhood neglect	2.1* (0.4)	3.4 (0.5)	32.1* (5.5)	59.5 (7.1)	23.9 (10.3)	19.7 (7.7)
Childhood physical abuse	3.2* (0.4)	4.8 (0.6)	33.8* (5.1)	56.6 (5.6)	22.3* (5.2)	48.5 (9.5)
Other qualifying trauma	2.2 (0.5)	2.7 (0.4)	18.7* (6.8)	31.8 (6.5)	12.7* (4.8)	33.4 (8.0)
Any trauma	60.7* (1.9)	51.2 (1.9)	8.2* (1.0)	20.4 (1.5)	…	…

Number of traumas

One	26.5 (1.5)	26.3 (1.7)				
Two	14.5 (0.9)	13.5 (0.9)				
Three	9.5 (0.9)	5.0 (0.6)				
Four or more	10.2 (0.8)	6.4 (0.6)				

[a]Prevalence of lifetime PTSD among respondents who ever experienced the trauma, whether or not the trauma was nominated as most upsetting.

[b]Prevalence of PTSD among those for whom the trauma was either their only or their "most upsetting."

*Gender difference significant at the 0.05 level, two-tailed test.

more likely than men to experience traumas with the highest magnitude of impact. Furthermore, women were significantly more likely than men to meet the criteria for PTSD when exposure to all traumas other than combat was considered. The combination of these influences—greater exposure to the higher-impact traumas and greater likelihood of developing PTSD once exposed—leads to the overall finding that women exposed to a trauma are more than twice as likely as men to develop PTSD (20.4% of women vs. 8.2% of men in the NCS sample).

The prevalences of PTSD associated with particular traumas in the subsamples of respondents who nominated those traumas as their only or their "most upsetting" were also examined (third set of columns in Table 2–2). With the exceptions of rape and combat exposure among the men and other qualifying traumas among the women, these proportions were smaller than those for respondents who had experienced a trauma that may or may not have been considered by them the most upsetting (second set of columns in Table 2–2). This could indicate that the risk of PTSD associated with any one event alone is usually less powerful than the lifetime risk of PTSD associated with a history of multiple events. However, because the NCS only assessed PTSD for one event, the issue of cumulative lifetime risk of PTSD after exposure to multiple traumatic events cannot be examined in more detail here.

We also examined the probability of having particular types of traumatic events in the subsample of respondents with a lifetime history of PTSD (Table 2–3), in contrast to the probability of having PTSD in the subsamples of respondents with different events as in Table 2–2. The events most commonly associated with PTSD among men were combat exposure (which occurred in 37.6% of PTSD cases and was the nominated event in 28.8% of cases) and witnessing someone being badly injured or killed (which occurred in 71.0% of cases and was the nominated event in 24.3%). Combat exposure is a fairly uncommon event (6.4% lifetime prevalence among men) associated with a high risk of PTSD (38.8%) (Table 2–2). Witnessing a bad injury or death, in comparison, is a much more common event (35.6% lifetime prevalence among men) associated with a low risk of PTSD (6.4%). Among women, the most common causes of PTSD were rape (which was reported in 42.1% of cases and nominated as most upsetting in 29.9% of cases) and sexual molestation (which was reported in 38.9% of cases and nominated as most upsetting in 19.1% of cases). Together, rape and molestation accounted for 49.0% of all cases of PTSD among women. The great importance of these events as causes of nearly half of all the PTSD reported by women derives from the combination of frequent occurrence (9.2% for rape and 12.3% for molestation) and substantial impact on PTSD (46.1% for rape and 26.4% for molestation).

The results concerning the types of traumatic experiences that lead to PTSD are relevant to a controversy concerning the DSM-IV criterion for PTSD that the trauma must be outside the range of usual human experience and of a type that would be markedly dis-

Table 2–3. Proportion of respondents with PTSD in the National Comorbidity Survey, by sex, reporting each trauma as the only one experienced or, if exposure was to more than one, the "most upsetting"

Trauma	Men % (SE)	Women % (SE)
Rape	5.4* (2.8)	29.9 (3.4)
Molestation	1.8* (0.7)	19.1 (3.1)
Physical attack	1.4* (0.6)	5.9 (1.6)
Combat	28.8 (6.1)	. . .
Shock	4.5 (1.4)	6.8 (1.2)
Threat w/weapon	2.5* (1.1)	7.7 (2.2)
Accident	12.1 (3.4)	5.1 (2.4)
Natural disaster w/fire	5.2 (2.5)	3.5 (2.3)
Witness	24.3* (4.8)	4.9 (1.1)
Childhood neglect	2.8 (1.1)	1.8 (0.7)
Childhood physical abuse	7.4 (2.0)	8.2 (2.9)
Other qualifying trauma	3.8 (1.6)	7.0 (2.1)
Any trauma	100.0 (. . .)	100.0 (. . .)

*Gender difference significant at the 0.05 level, two-tailed test.

tressing to almost anyone. Our results are consistent with recent research showing that virtually all of the qualifying events for PTSD are quite common (Kilpatrick and Resnick 1992), and none is such that the great majority of people exposed to it develop PTSD. Also, there is enormous variability in the risk of PTSD across traumatic events. Furthermore, events that are traumatic in one sector of the population may not be traumatic in another. For example, men in the NCS sample were nearly twice as likely as women to report having been seriously physically attacked or assaulted (11.1% vs. 6.9%) (Table 2–2). Yet this type of event was 15 times more likely to provoke PTSD among women than among men (21.3% vs. 1.8%). Subgroup differences such as this make it very difficult to categorize stressful events neatly into those that are traumatic and those that are not traumatic (March 1992).

Demographic Correlates of Trauma Exposure and PTSD

We examined the associations between lifetime PTSD and a number of sociodemographic correlates for the NCS sample with logistic regression analyses (Table 2–4).

Sex

Consistent with our earlier results, women had a significantly higher lifetime prevalence of PTSD compared with men. This higher prevalence was found despite the fact that women were significantly less likely than men to report a trauma. The greater risk of PTSD among women in this sample can be accounted for in large part by the fact that women were much more likely than men to develop PTSD once they were exposed to a trauma. This greater vulnerability derives in part from the finding that traumas experienced by women had a higher magnitude of impact than those experienced by men (i.e., odds ratio [OR] for trauma subsample smaller when type of trauma controlled). However, women were much more vulnerable than men even when sex differences in the types of trauma experienced were controlled (i.e., OR for trauma subsample still significant after types of trauma controlled).

Table 2–4. Disaggregated analysis of sociodemographic correlates of lifetime posttraumatic stress disorder (PTSD) in a National Comorbidity Survey sample

	Risk of PTSD OR (95% CI)	Risk of trauma OR (95% CI)	Risk of PTSD in trauma subsample OR (95% CI)	Risk of PTSD in trauma sub-sample with type of trauma controlled[a] OR (95% CI)
Sex				
Male	1.00 (. . .)	1.00 (. . .)	1.00 (. . .)	1.00 (. . .)
Female	2.24* (1.63, 3.07)	0.68* (0.55, 0.84)	2.89* (2.09, 3.99)	2.49* (1.72, 3.61)
Age, years (females)				
15–24	1.00 (. . .)	1.00 (. . .)	1.00 (. . .)	1.00 (. . .)
25–34	1.10 (0.80, 1.51)	1.06 (0.80, 1.40)	1.05 (0.71, 1.55)	0.97 (0.62, 1.51)
35–44	1.04 (0.70, 1.54)	1.51* (1.15, 1.99)	0.82 (0.54, 1.23)	0.81 (0.46, 1.41)
45+	0.86 (0.51, 1.46)	1.09 (0.78, 1.53)	0.79 (0.45, 1.40)	0.80 (0.49, 1.32)
Age, years (males)				
15–24	1.00 (. . .)	1.00 (. . .)	1.00 (. . .)	1.00 (. . .)
25–34	2.09* (1.13, 3.86)	1.41* (1.00, 1.96)	1.84 (0.97, 3.50)	1.63 (0.79, 3.36)
35–44	1.82 (0.76, 4.37)	1.72* (1.22, 2.42)	1.48 (0.61, 3.55)	0.65 (0.25, 1.67)
45+	2.87* (1.36, 6.08)	2.23* (1.42, 3.52)	2.18* (1.00, 4.75)	1.16 (0.42, 3.16)

(continued)

Table 2–4. Disaggregated analysis of sociodemographic correlates of lifetime posttraumatic stress disorder (PTSD) in a National Comorbidity Survey sample (*continued*)

	Risk of PTSD	Risk of trauma	Risk of PTSD in trauma subsample	Risk of PTSD in trauma subsample with type of trauma controlled[a]
	OR (95% CI)	OR (95% CI)	OR (95% CI)	OR (95% CI)
Race				
White	1.00 (. . .)	1.00 (. . .)	1.00 (. . .)	1.00 (. . .)
Black	1.07 (0.65, 1.78)	0.63* (0.46, 0.89)	1.40 (0.82, 2.39)	1.23 (0.66, 2.29)
Hispanic	1.29 (0.73, 2.27)	1.06 (0.74, 1.54)	1.27 (0.70, 2.33)	0.95 (0.45, 2.01)
Other	1.15 (0.61, 2.16)	0.62* (0.41, 0.94)	1.54 (0.71, 3.33)	2.17 (0.90, 5.19)
Education, grades[b]				
0–11	1.83* (1.11, 3.03)	0.75 (0.50, 1.14)	2.18* (1.26, 3.78)	2.69* (1.41, 5.11)
12	1.44 (0.88, 2.37)	0.67* (0.51, 0.87)	1.80* (1.06, 3.06)	2.09* (1.14, 3.83)
13–15	1.60 (0.93, 2.76)	0.98 (0.72, 1.35)	1.65 (0.96, 2.84)	1.88* (1.03, 3.45)
16+	1.00 (. . .)	1.00 (. . .)	1.00 (. . .)	1.00 (. . .)

Income, dollars (thousands)[b]				
00–19	1.94* (1.03, 3.65)	0.91 (0.62, 1.32)	2.12* (1.10, 4.12)	2.10* (1.09, 4.04)
20–34	1.49 (0.79, 2.82)	0.72* (0.53, 0.99)	1.80 (0.89, 3.63)	2.08* (1.06, 4.07)
35–69	1.04 (0.56, 1.91)	0.88 (0.60, 1.30)	1.10 (0.58, 2.09)	1.19 (0.63, 2.25)
70+	1.00 (. . .)	1.00 (. . .)	1.00 (. . .)	1.00 (. . .)
Marital status (females)				
Never married	1.00 (. . .)	1.00 (. . .)	1.00 (. . .)	1.00 (. . .)
Married	1.27 (0.77, 2.10)	1.02 (0.73, 1.42)	1.33 (0.78, 2.26)	1.20 (0.76, 1.91)
Previously married	2.86* (1.48, 5.53)	1.35 (0.83, 2.21)	2.93* (1.14, 6.08)	2.59* (1.33, 5.06)
Marital status (males)				
Never married	1.00 (. . .)	1.00 (. . .)	1.00 (. . .)	1.00 (. . .)
Married	3.82* (1.64, 8.87)	1.14 (0.79, 1.63)	3.56* (1.62, 7.82)	3.21* (1.43, 7.86)
Previously married	6.00* (1.73, 20.79)	1.60 (0.87, 2.93)	5.11* (1.39, 18.71)	3.47 (0.96, 15.04)
Region				
Northeast	1.36 (0.95, 1.94)	1.01 (0.69, 1.46)	1.38 (0.91, 2.08)	1.39 (0.83, 2.30)
South	1.34 (0.99, 1.82)	1.04 (0.74, 1.46)	1.34 (0.97, 1.85)	1.41 (0.98, 2.21)
Midwest	1.00 (. . .)	1.00 (. . .)	1.00 (. . .)	1.00 (. . .)
West	1.87* (1.32, 2.70)	1.92* (1.37, 2.69)	1.45* (1.03, 2.05)	1.38 (0.85, 2.20)

(continued)

Table 2–4. Disaggregated analysis of sociodemographic correlates of lifetime posttraumatic stress disorder (PTSD) in a National Comorbidity Survey sample *(continued)*

Urbanicity				
Metro	1.09 (0.71, 1.69)	1.13 (0.79, 1.59)	1.03 (0.69, 1.55)	0.82 (0.53, 1.27)
Other metro	0.93 (0.60, 1.45)	1.07 (0.66, 1.71)	0.89 (0.60, 1.33)	0.69 (0.47, 1.02)
Rural	1.00 (. . .)	1.00 (. . .)	1.00 (. . .)	1.00 (. . .)

Note. OR = odds ratio; CI = confidence interval. The ORs in Column 1 describe the zero-order associations between each demographic variable and PTSD in the sample as a whole. The results in the rest of the table decompose these total associations into components based on the relationships of the demographic variable with exposure to at least one trauma (Column 2), with PTSD in the subsample of respondents exposed to at least one trauma (Column 3), and with the net associations in the subsample of respondents exposed to at least one trauma after the type of trauma experienced was controlled (Column 4). If the association of a particular demographic variable with PTSD is the result of its being associated with higher-impact traumas, the ORs in Column 3 will be larger than the ORs in Column 4.

[a]ORs reported in this column are based on multivariate models in which a series of dummy variables to define type of most upsetting/only trauma were introduced as control variables.

[b]The education and income models are based on restricted samples that exclude students.

*OR significant at the 0.05 level, two-tailed test.

Age

Because the relationship between age and lifetime prevalence of PTSD differed by sex, we estimated the ORs associated with age separately for men and women (Table 2–4). Among women, there was no significant overall association between age and PTSD, and there was evidence of only a modest increase in lifetime risk of exposure to a trauma with age. Nor were there any significant differences in risk of PTSD after exposure to a trauma among the different age groups. Further analysis of this pattern in terms of age at onset showed significant intercohort variation in exposure: women in more recent cohorts were significantly more likely than those in older cohorts to have experienced traumas during their teens or early twenties. In comparison, no evidence of intercohort variation in risk of PTSD after trauma exposure was found. Among men, in comparison, there was a substantial positive association between age and PTSD because of greater risk of exposure, but there was no evidence of intercohort variation in either trauma exposure or risk of PTSD after trauma exposure.

Race

No significant overall association between race and lifetime PTSD was found (Table 2–4). However, more detailed analyses showed that this lack of association was due to opposite-sign trends. Although "Blacks" and "Other" minorities (mostly Asians and Native Americans) were significantly less likely than "Whites" and "Hispanics" to experience a trauma (column 2 in Table 2–4), there was a trend for blacks and other minorities to be more likely than whites or Hispanics to develop PTSD once they are exposed to a trauma (column 3 in Table 2–4). The comparative advantage of low exposure and the comparative disadvantage of high vulnerability to PTSD after exposure cancelled each other out to yield the nonsignificant association found in the overall estimate for risk of PTSD (column 1 in Table 2–4). More detailed analyses showed that these results cannot be explained by controlling for income and education differences among these subsamples.

Education

The results concerning education presented in Table 2–4 are estimates after current students in the sample were eliminated from consideration. The sample was restricted in this way to avoid combining young people who were still in the process of completing their education (e.g., 15-year-old respondents in ninth grade) with older respondents who had dropped out of school at an early age (e.g., adult respondents who had dropped out of school in ninth grade). There was a significant negative association between education and lifetime PTSD among the remaining respondents in the sample. This association can be attributed to the fact that education was negatively associated with vulnerability to PTSD rather than with exposure to trauma (as can be seen from the ORs in columns 2–4 in Table 2–4).

Income

Following the same logic as was used in the education analysis, we eliminated current students from the sample before examining the relationship between income and PTSD. We found a significant negative association between income and lifetime PTSD among the remaining respondents in the sample (column 3 in Table 2–4). It is plausible to infer from this finding that low income is associated with high exposure to trauma. However, as the results in column 2 of Table 2–4 show, no such association was found. Instead, the higher prevalence of PTSD among low-income respondents in this sample is attributable to greater vulnerability to PTSD once exposure to a trauma has taken place. Middle-income respondents also had an elevated vulnerability to PTSD compared with respondents in the highest income category (column 4). This finding is masked in the data for the overall estimate for risk of PTSD (column 1) because middle-income respondents were less likely than high-income respondents to experience a trauma.

Marital Status

Lifetime PTSD was significantly more prevalent among the previously married than among the currently married for both men and women, when age was controlled (columns 3 and 4 in Table 2–4). Furthermore, among men, but not women, PTSD was significantly more prevalent among the currently married than among the never married, when age was controlled. As shown in Table 2–4, these associations resulted largely from a combination of significantly elevated probabilities of PTSD among respondents exposed to trauma rather than from differential lifetime probabilities of trauma exposure.

Region

Respondents in the Midwest had the lowest lifetime prevalence of PTSD, whereas those in the West had the highest (Table 2–4). The high prevalence in the West was the result of a twofold higher exposure to trauma compared with other parts of the country (column 2 in Table 2–4). The low prevalence in the Midwest was attributable to a lower vulnerability to PTSD once exposure to a trauma has taken place than in other parts of the country (column 3 in Table 2–4).

Urbanicity

No significant association between urbanicity and PTSD was found, either in the gross analysis of risk of PTSD (column 1 in Table 2–4) or in analyses controlling for differences in overall exposure and type of trauma exposure (columns 3 and 4).

In addition to the bivariate analyses reported in Table 2–4, parallel multivariate analyses were carried out to examine the associations of all the significant variables in the table. The results yielded coefficients quite similar to those in Table 2–4, with the exception that the simultaneous control for both education and income led to the disappearance of the significant associations involving both variables. It is noteworthy that "Blacks" and "Other" minorities were still found in this multivariate analysis to be significantly less likely to experience a trauma than "Whites," even after all other demographic variables were controlled. This could represent a substantive finding or a methodological artifact arising from differences in the accuracy of recall or in the interpretation of vaguely defined terms such as "assault" or "abuse." Research is needed to develop procedures that minimize the problems of both recall bias (Kessler et al., in press) and misunderstanding due to use of vaguely defined terms to describe traumatic situations (Kilpatrick and Resnick 1992) in an effort to distinguish correlations that are substantive from those that are artifactual.

Effects of Comorbidity

A consistently significant cross-sectional relationship was found between lifetime PTSD and lifetime history of most other NCS/DSM-III-R disorders among both men and women in the NCS sample (Kessler et al. 1995). Among respondents with a lifetime history of PTSD, 88.3% of the men and 79.0% of the women reported a lifetime history of at least one other disorder. These results are consistent with those from a number of previous studies in both treatment samples (Davidson et al. 1985; Green et al. 1989; Sierles et al. 1983) and general population samples (Centers for Disease Control 1988; Kilpatrick and Resnick 1992; Shore et al. 1989) in showing that PTSD is highly comorbid with a number of other disorders.

We also investigated the time-lagged effects of other disorders as risk factors for subsequent development of PTSD. To study these effects, we estimated a discrete-time survival model in which prior histories of other disorders were treated as time-varying predictors of first onset of PTSD (Efron 1988). The results are reported in Tables 2–5 (for male respondents) and 2–6 (for female respondents). The ORs in Column 1 of the tables describe the overall associations of other disorders with subsequent PTSD. The vast majority of these ORs are greater than 1.0, which indicates that prior histories of most other disorders were associated with increased risk of subsequent PTSD. The effect of having at least one prior disorder, no matter what disorder, was more powerful than

Table 2–5. Earlier onset of other disorders as predictors of posttraumatic stress disorder (PTSD) among men in a National Comorbidity Survey sample

	Risk of PTSD in total sample	Risk of trauma	Risk of PTSD in trauma subsample	Risk of PTSD in trauma sub-sample with type of trauma controlled[a]
	OR (95% CI)	OR (95% CI)	OR (95% CI)	OR (95% CI)
Mood disorders				
MDE	5.25* (2.49, 11.08)	1.03 (0.70, 1.50)	3.93* (1.36, 11.40)	4.14* (1.41, 12.12)
Dysthymia	2.06 (0.80, 5.36)	1.67 (0.85, 3.26)	1.80 (0.61, 5.28)	1.74 (0.55, 5.55)
Mania	2.30* (1.03, 5.13)	1.02 (0.70, 1.49)	. . .	. . .
Any mood disorder	5.87* (2.55, 13.50)	1.38* (1.01, 1.88)	4.05* (1.65, 9.94)	3.63* (1.56, 8.44)
Anxiety disorders				
GAD	0.45 (0.10, 2.10)	0.82 (0.57, 1.18)	1.34 (0.19, 9.51)	1.46 (0.12, 17.56)
Panic disorder	1.62 (0.60, 4.38)	1.53 (0.61, 3.81)	1.87 (0.43, 8.21)	2.70 (0.35, 20.87)
Simple phobia	3.86* (2.19, 6.80)	1.32* (1.05, 1.66)	3.55* (1.58, 7.99)	4.46* (1.71, 11.64)
Social phobia	0.69 (0.37, 1.30)	0.95 (0.79, 1.14)	0.69 (0.36, 1.33)	0.90 (0.48, 1.70)
Agoraphobia	2.46* (1.41, 4.28)	1.59* (1.20, 2.11)	1.40* (0.41, 4.80)	1.01 (0.30, 3.42)
Any anxiety disorder	2.37* (1.50, 3.75)	1.20* (1.03, 1.39)	2.01* (1.22, 3.30)	2.70* (1.56, 4.67)

(continued)

Table 2–5. Earlier onset of other disorders as predictors of posttraumatic stress disorder (PTSD) among men in a National Comorbidity Survey sample *(continued)*

	Risk of PTSD in total sample OR (95% CI)	Risk of trauma OR (95% CI)	Risk of PTSD in trauma subsample OR (95% CI)	Risk of PTSD in trauma sub-sample with type of trauma controlled[a] OR (95% CI)
Substance use disorders				
Alcohol abuse/dependence	1.69 (0.84, 3.41)	1.45* (1.23, 1.70)	0.89 (0.40, 1.99)	1.16 (0.52, 2.57)
Drug abuse/dependence	1.24 (0.60, 2.55)	1.47* (1.14, 1.90)	0.95 (0.33, 2.75)	0.92 (0.37, 2.32)
Any substance use disorder	2.26* (1.38, 3.70)	1.65* (1.38, 1.98)	0.97 (0.53, 1.77)	1.41 (0.77, 2.58)
Other disorder				
Conduct disorder	1.75 (0.91, 3.37)	1.44* (1.20, 1.73)	1.35 (0.62, 2.96)	1.67 (0.75, 3.72)
Any disorder[b]				
No Dx	1.00 (. . .)	1.00 (. . .)	1.00 (. . .)	1.00 (. . .)
One Dx	4.95* (3.50, 7.01)	1.66* (1.53, 1.80)	1.80* (1.06, 3.08)	3.34* (1.69, 6.58)
Two Dx	9.35* (4.73, 18.50)	2.11* (1.67, 2.66)	3.90* (2.22, 6.86)	4.30* (2.02, 9.15)
Three or more Dx	22.20* (9.82, 48.98)	2.82* (1.98, 4.03)	5.15* (1.56, 16.97)	7.50* (2.86, 19.62)

Note. OR = odds ratio; CI = confidence interval; MDE = major depressive episode; GAD = generalized anxiety disorder; Dx = diagnosis (diagnoses).

[a]ORs reported in this column are based on multivariate models in which a series of dummy variables to define type of most upsetting/only trauma were introduced as control variables.

[b]Excluding disorders with odds ratios less than 1.5.

*OR significant at the 0.05 level, two-tailed test.

Table 2–6. Early onset of other disorders as predictors of PTSD among women in a National Comorbidity Survey sample

	Risk of PTSD in total sample	Risk of trauma	Risk of PTSD in trauma subsample	Risk of PTSD in trauma subsample with type of trauma controlled[a]
	OR (95% CI)	OR (95% CI)	OR (95% CI)	OR (95% CI)
Mood disorders				
MDE	3.29* (1.86, 5.80)	1.79* (1.41, 2.28)	1.43 (0.89, 2.29)	1.84* (1.12, 3.05)
Dysthymia	2.39* (1.00, 5.80)	1.18 (0.94, 1.48)	1.96 (0.93, 4.14)	1.61 (0.67, 3.89)
Mania	1.19 (0.29, 4.94)	1.15 (0.61, 2.16)	· · ·	· · ·
Any mood disorder	3.50* (1.86, 6.57)	1.89* (1.57, 2.27)	1.49* (0.93, 2.41)	1.72* (1.00, 2.64)
Anxiety disorders				
GAD	0.87 (0.40, 1.90)	0.97 (0.65, 1.43)	0.87 (0.23, 3.21)	0.80 (0.20, 3.19)
Panic disorder	0.99 (0.36, 2.70)	1.57 (0.74, 3.32)	0.87 (0.19, 4.00)	0.61 (0.16, 2.28)
Simple phobia	1.31 (0.81, 2.11)	1.05 (0.84, 1.31)	1.32 (0.78, 2.22)	1.43 (0.82, 2.50)
Social phobia	1.61 (0.98, 2.65)	1.30* (1.04, 1.59)	1.16 (0.75, 1.79)	1.57 (0.92, 2.68)
Agoraphobia	1.57 (0.74, 3.33)	1.00 (0.73, 1.38)	1.79 (0.71, 4.51)	1.36 (0.56, 3.28)
Any anxiety disorder	2.00* (1.36, 2.90)	1.32* (1.11, 1.56)	1.54* (1.03, 2.29)	1.63* (1.01, 2.64)

(continued)

Table 2–6. Early onset of other disorders as predictors of PTSD among women in a National Comorbidity Survey sample *(continued)*

	Risk of PTSD in total sample	Risk of trauma	Risk of PTSD in trauma subsample	Risk of PTSD in trauma subsample with type of trauma controlled[a]
	OR (95% CI)	OR (95% CI)	OR (95% CI)	OR (95% CI)
Substance use disorders				
Alcohol abuse/dependence	1.02 (0.46, 2.29)	1.42* (1.15, 1.74)	0.59 (0.28, 1.25)	0.67 (0.33, 1.37)
Drug abuse/dependence	2.72 (0.70, 10.60)	1.47* (1.06, 2.03)	1.93 (0.85, 4.35)	1.52 (0.69, 3.35)
Any substance use disorder	2.15* (1.16, 3.98)	1.65* (1.22, 2.24)	1.21 (0.88, 1.68)	1.19 (0.76, 1.86)
Other disorder				
Conduct disorder	2.22 (0.91, 5.38)	1.32* (0.93, 1.89)	1.49 (0.53, 4.19)	1.88 (0.72, 4.90)
Any disorder[b]				
No Dx	1.00 (. . .)	1.00 (. . .)	1.00 (. . .)	1.00 (. . .)
One Dx	3.43* (2.53, 4.66)	1.70* (1.49, 1.94)	1.40 (0.91, 2.15)	1.71* (1.07, 2.71)
Two Dx	4.74* (2.86, 7.86)	2.04* (1.62, 2.58)	1.84* (1.01, 3.36)	2.53* (1.31, 4.87)
Three or more Dx	13.26* (6.37, 27.60)	3.04* (2.10, 4.39)	5.05* (1.69, 15.07)	5.27* (1.75, 15.87)

Note. OR = odds ratio; CI = confidence interval; MDE = major depressive episode; GAD = generalized anxiety disorder; Dx = diagnosis (diagnoses).

[a]ORs reported in this column are based on multivariate models in which a series of dummy variables to define type of most upsetting/only trauma were introduced as control variables.

[b]Excluding disorders with odds ratios less than 1.5.

the effect of having nearly any of the specific disorders. Furthermore, the effect of having multiple prior disorders was greater than the effect of having only one prior disorder. This was especially true among men.

The data in the remaining columns of Table 2–5 and 2–6 represent a disaggregation of the overall associations presented in column 1 of those tables. The results in column 2 in both tables show that the summary measures of any mood disorder, any anxiety disorder, any substance use disorder, and, among men, conduct disorder are all associated with greater risk of exposure to subsequent trauma. The results in column 3 show that among those respondents exposed to trauma, any mood disorder and any anxiety disorder are both associated with greater vulnerability to PTSD. The predictive effects of having multiple prior disorders are consistently larger than those of having nearly any of the specific disorders on both exposure to trauma and subsequent onset of PTSD.

In the analyses reported in Tables 2–5 and 2–6, age at onset of PTSD was defined as the age associated with the onset of PTSD that resulted from the respondent's "most upsetting" or only traumatic event. Respondents who reported the lifetime occurrence of multiple events might have had another episode of PTSD at an earlier age, in which case the estimated associations between "earlier" disorders (i.e., those earlier than the "most upsetting" event) and subsequent PTSD might actually represent effects of earlier PTSD. We could not evaluate this possibility definitively with these data because the NCS assessed PTSD for only one event per person.

A partial evaluation was carried out, however, by replicating the analyses used to generate the results that estimate the effects of disorders with onset prior to the respondent's first trauma (rather than with onset prior to the "most upsetting" trauma) on PTSD as of the year of the first trauma. This replication was carried out based on the conservative assumption (from the perspective of estimating the effects of earlier disorders on subsequent PTSD) that all respondents who developed PTSD in response to their "most upsetting" event also developed it earlier in life in response to their first trauma, and on the assumption that respondents who did not develop PTSD in response to their "most upsetting" trauma also failed to do so in response to their earliest (and less upsetting) trauma. As shown in Table 2–7, affective disorders, anxiety disorders, and substance use disorders that occurred prior to the respondent's first trauma were all significantly associated with risk of subsequent PTSD among both men and women.

The partial analysis that yielded the results in Tables 2–5 through 2–7 was based on the assumption that the effects of prior disorders on PTSD are constant over time. Further analysis showed that this is not true: the ORs become progressively less powerful with an increase in time since the onset of the predictor disorders. Therefore, the results in Tables 2–5 through 2–7 are, in effect, averages of time-variant effects that are strongest in the year after onset of the predictor disorder and become progressively weaker over time. In addition, we found that the cross-sectional ORs—the ORs between risk of onset of PTSD and of other disorders in the same year—were uniformly very large.

More detailed examination of this last finding uncovered a number of respondents who reported a number of different disorders that all started in the same year as their PTSD. A prototypical case involved a young woman who reported being raped at the age of 15 and having had her first panic attack and developed social phobia, agoraphobia, major depression, generalized anxiety disorder, and PTSD all at this same age. Clearly, this should not be considered a case of "comorbidity" among several distinct disorders, but rather a complex reaction to a traumatic experience that our current nosological system is incapable of describing other than by artificially characterizing the reaction in terms of comorbidity. It is important for researchers both to recognize that cases of this sort do exist and to control for the strong clustering created by these cases in investigations of comorbidity of PTSD with other disorders.

Importance of Randomly Selected Traumas

Because in the NCS we assessed PTSD for only one event per person, the event-specific analyses described in the preceding sections focused on the subsample of events that were rated "most upset-

Table 2–7. Onset of other disorders as of the age of the respondent at first trauma as predictors of PTSD in a National Comorbidity Survey sample

	Men OR (95% CI)	Women OR (95% CI)
Mood disorders		
MDE	4.51* (1.82, 11.19)	3.03* (1.77, 5.19)
Dysthymia	0.41 (0.10, 1.70)	2.00 (0.83, 4.81)
Mania	. . .	. . .
Any mood disorder	3.22* (1.31, 7.91)	2.52* (1.42, 4.47)
Anxiety disorders		
GAD	. . .	0.53 (0.14, 1.97)
Panic disorder	1.54 (0.10, 24.25)	0.40 (0.07, 2.15)
Simple phobia	4.45* (2.32, 8.55)	1.89* (1.17, 3.06)
Social phobia	0.98 (0.52, 1.86)	1.52 (0.98, 2.37)
Agoraphobia	2.65 (0.86, 8.12)	1.20 (0.42, 3.39)
Any anxiety disorder	2.79* (1.58, 4.92)	1.98* (1.35, 2.88)
Substance use disorders		
Alcohol abuse/dependence	2.06 (0.76, 5.59)	1.16 (0.34, 3.89)
Drug abuse/dependence	2.33 (0.63, 8.74)	3.30 (0.90, 12.06)
Any substance use disorder	3.84* (1.64, 9.03)	2.35* (1.17, 4.74)
Other disorder		
Conduct disorder	1.87 (0.64, 5.40)	2.25 (0.60, 8.41)
Any disorder[a]		
No Dx	1.00 (. . .)	1.00 (. . .)
One Dx	5.59* (3.13, 10.00)	2.81* (1.94, 4.07)
Two Dx	6.08* (1.97, 18.80)	5.22* (2.92, 9.33)
Three or more Dx	24.06* (9.59, 60.34)	9.74* (2.53, 37.55)

Note. OR = odds ratio; CI = confidence interval; MDE = major depressive episode; GAD = generalized anxiety disorder; Dx = diagnosis (diagnoses).
[a]Excluding disorders with odds ratios less than 1.5.
*OR significant at the 0.05 level, two-tailed test.

ting" by respondents who had experienced two or more lifetime traumas. With this approach there is the potential for an overestimation of the effects of particular events. For example, whereas 65.0% of the subsample of men who reported that being raped was either their only or their "most upsetting" lifetime trauma developed PTSD after that event, a much smaller proportion (46.4%) of the larger group of all men who reported having been raped (whether or not it was their only or "most upsetting" trauma) reported lifetime PTSD associated with their "most upsetting" trauma. The most plausible way to interpret this discrepancy is to assume that the rapes nominated as "most upsetting" were more traumatizing than those not nominated as "most upsetting."

The only way to correct this bias is to assess each respondent's entire trauma history and the PTSD associated either with each lifetime trauma or with a randomly selected subsample of lifetime traumas. A complete assessment of PTSD for each trauma experienced by each respondent in a community survey would be a formidable task because of the large number of traumas involved. The results in Table 2–2 show that more than 10% of men and 6% of women in the NCS reported four or more types of lifetime traumas, some of which involved multiple occurrences (e.g., being in two or more natural disasters at different times in their life). In some cases, a complete assessment of trauma history for a single respondent would involve an assessment of PTSD associated with each of as many as two dozen separate traumas. Given the enormous burden on the respondent that would be imposed by this task, assessment of a randomly selected subsample of lifetime traumas is more practical.

Two of the present authors (R.C.K. and N.B.) created an interview schedule to assess PTSD for a randomly selected trauma. We recently administered this interview to a representative community sample of people in the Detroit metropolitan area. The selection of a "random" trauma required a complete enumeration of trauma exposure. This turned out to be a more complex operation than we originally realized because we had to enumerate not only each type of trauma experienced by each respondent but also the number of times each type of trauma had been experienced. This process was especially challenging when a respondent reported exposure to numerous linked traumas, as in the case of the woman who reported having been repeatedly raped throughout her childhood by a stepbrother. A special data collection strategy was developed to deal with such cases by recording linked traumas as special cases of "single" events that were categorized by age at onset and duration of exposure.

We assessed PTSD for both one "random" trauma (i.e., one trauma randomly selected from all lifetime traumas for each respondent who reported exposure to more than one lifetime trauma) and the "most upsetting" trauma for each respondent. Preliminary analyses, which are all we have completed to date, show that many results regarding patterns and risk factors for PTSD differ substantially depending on whether we study randomly selected or "most upsetting" traumas. For example, the estimated conditional risk of PTSD after trauma exposure is much lower, and the intertrauma variation in PTSD risk is much greater, when we focus on "random" traumas rather than "most upsetting" traumas. Results based on previous epidemiological surveys that focused on "most upsetting" traumas, including those from the NCS, are seriously limited in terms of allowing one to draw valid inferences about risk factors for PTSD. This limitation includes bias not only in estimates of risk factor effects but also in estimates of basic risk assessments such as the conditional probability of PTSD given trauma exposure and the differential risk of PTSD across types of trauma.

To say that we focused on "randomly selected" traumas in this new survey is not to say that the traumas we studied occurred randomly with respect to prior characteristics of the respondents who experienced them. To the contrary, our findings show quite clearly that a number of sociodemographic factors and prior psychiatric disorders predict trauma exposure. This is equally true of the traumas we selected at random and those nominated by respondents as "most upsetting." However, by assessing PTSD for traumas selected by us at random from all the traumas each respondent ever experienced, rather than allowing the respondent to talk only about the trauma that he or she experienced as "most upsetting," we were able to see the effects of more typical and less severe traumas than those assessed in previous general population epidemiological studies.

Our finding that typical traumas are much less likely to lead to PTSD than traumas nominated by respondents as "most upsetting" raises an important question about the assumption in the DSM system that the diagnosis of PTSD should be made only for reactions to events that are outside of the range of usual human experience and that would be considered traumatic by most people. We found that most of the events recognized by the DSM system as qualifying events for a diagnosis of PTSD are actually quite common rather than outside the range of usual normal experience. We found that none of these traumas is so powerful that exposure typically leads to PTSD. Thus, we believe that future general population research should broaden the range of stressful experiences evaluated in the context of PTSD beyond those currently defined as qualifying in the DSM system. In doing this, it will be impossible to assess PTSD for each such event because most people experience a number of potentially stressful events at some time in their lives. Therefore, we advocate the complete enumeration of lifetime major traumas and the complete enumeration of other stressor events over a shorter recall period, followed by an evaluation of PTSD associated with a randomly selected subsample of these experiences for each respondent. It is important that this be done in a representative sample. In addition, it would be useful if probes were included to learn something about variation in objective stressor characteristics. Analysis of such a data array would be a major step forward in documenting empirically the range of stressful experiences that lead to pathological stress response syndromes and more clearly investigating individual differences in stress reactivity over a wide range of the stress severity spectrum.

Conclusion

In this chapter, we have presented data from the National Comorbidity Survey on epidemiological risk factors for posttraumatic stress disorder. Considerable variation was found in risk of

PTSD across trauma types. This is consistent with the results of previous research on between-trauma variation (Kilpatrick and Resnick 1992; March 1992), but inconsistent with recent studies that failed to find differential risk of PTSD within trauma types associated with severity of the stressor (Feinstein and Dolan 1991; Perry et al. 1992). A number of sociodemographic predictors of PTSD were documented, most of them associated much less with trauma exposure than with risk of PTSD after exposure. Prior histories of other DSM disorders were found to be very powerful predictors of PTSD. Mood and anxiety disorders were less powerful predictors of trauma exposure than of PTSD after exposure. Addictive disorders and conduct disorder, in comparison, were stronger predictors of trauma exposure than of PTSD after exposure.

A weakness of the NCS is that PTSD was evaluated for only one self-nominated "most upsetting" lifetime trauma even though the majority of respondents reported experiencing more than one trauma in their lifetimes. Some selective focus of this sort was required because the number of traumas reported was so large that we could not evaluate relation to PTSD separately for each one. However, the focus on an atypical trauma was unfortunate, in retrospect, in that it made it impossible either to draw valid inferences about the impact of typical traumas or to evaluate the impact of factors such as age at trauma exposure or prior history of other traumas on PTSD risk. As described above, we suggest that future general population studies of PTSD attempt to carry out a complete trauma exposure enumeration and then select not only the "most upsetting" trauma but also one or more "random" traumas for each respondent to evaluate for PTSD. This procedure, which we implemented in a survey carried out after the NCS, is likely to yield much more useful information about typical trauma effects and might even find evidence of different risk factors than those found in studies of most "upsetting traumas." It would also be very useful to carry out a longitudinal general population survey of trauma exposure and PTSD in order to remove the problem of retrospective recall bias that clouds interpretation of epidemiological risk factors in cross-sectional surveys. We hope to address this problem in a planned reinterview survey of the NCS respondents.

References

American Psychiatric Association: Diagnostic and Statistical Manual of Mental Disorders, 3rd Edition. Washington, DC, American Psychiatric Association, 1980

American Psychiatric Association: Diagnostic and Statistical Manual of Mental Disorders, 3rd Edition, Revised. Washington, DC, American Psychiatric Association, 1987

American Psychiatric Association: Diagnostic and Statistical Manual of Mental Disorders, 4th Edition. Washington, DC, American Psychiatric Association, 1994

Breslau N, Davis GC, Andreski P, et al: Traumatic events and posttraumatic stress disorder in an urban population of young adults. Arch Gen Psychiatry 48:216–222, 1991

Burgess AW, Holstrum L: The rape trauma syndrome. Am J Psychiatry 131:981–986, 1974

Centers for Disease Control: Health status of Vietnam veterans: psychosocial characteristics. JAMA 259:2701–2707, 1988

Croyle RT, Loftus EF: Improving episode memory performance of survey respondents, in Questions About Questions: Inquiries Into the Cognitive Bases of Surveys. Edited by Tanur JM. New York, Russell Sage Foundation, 1992, pp 95–101

Davidson JRT, Swartz M, Stork M, et al: A diagnostic and family study of posttraumatic stress disorder. Am J Psychiatry 142:90–93, 1985

Davidson JRT, Kudler HS, Saunders WB, et al: Symptom and morbidity patterns in World War II and Vietnam veterans with posttraumatic stress disorder. Compr Psychiatry 31:1162–1170, 1990

Davidson JRT, Hughes D, Blazer D, et al: Posttraumatic stress disorder in the community: an epidemiological study. Psychol Med 21:1–19, 1991

Efron B: Logistic regression, survival analysis, and the Kaplan-Meier Curve. Journal of the American Statistical Association 70:414–425, 1988

Endicott J, Spitzer RL: A diagnostic interview: the Schedule for Affective Disorders and Schizophrenia. Arch Gen Psychiatry 35:837–844, 1978

Feinstein A, Dolan R: Predictors of post-traumatic stress disorder following physical trauma: an examination of the stressor criterion. Psychol Med 21:85–91, 1991

Frank E, Anderson BP: Psychiatric disorders in rape victims: past history and current symptomatology. Compr Psychiatry 28:77–82, 1987

Freud S: Introduction to Psycho-Analysis and the War Neuroses (1919), in The Standard Edition of the Complete Psychological Works of Sigmund Freud, Vol 18. Translated and edited by Strachey J. London, Hogarth Press, 1955, pp 205–215

Goenjian AK, Najarian LM, Pynoos RS, et al: Posttraumatic stress disorder in elderly and younger adults after the 1988 earthquake in Armenia. Am J Psychiatry 151:895–901, 1994

Green BL: Psychosocial research in traumatic stress: an update. Journal of Traumatic Stress 7:341–362, 1994

Green BL, Lindy JD, Grace MC, et al: Multiple diagnosis in posttraumatic stress disorder: the role of war stressors. J Nerv Ment Dis 177:329–335, 1989

Grinker K, Spiegel S: Men Under Stress. Philadelphia, PA, Blakiston, 1945

Helzer JE, Robins LN, McEvoy L: Post-traumatic stress disorder in the general population. N Engl J Med 317:1630–1634, 1987

Horowitz MJ: Stress Response Syndromes. New York, Jason Aronson, 1976

Keller MB, Lavori PW, Nielsen E: SCALUP (SCID plus SADS-L). Providence, RI, Butler Hospital, Department of Psychiatry, 1987

Kessler RC, Wethington E: The reliability of life event reports in a community survey. Psychol Med 21:723–738, 1991

Kessler RC, McGonagle KA, Zhao S, et al: Lifetime and 12-month prevalence of DSM-III-R psychiatric disorders in the United States: results from the National Comorbidity Survey. Arch Gen Psychiatry 51:8–19, 1994

Kessler RC, Sonnega A, Bromet E, et al: Posttraumatic stress disorder in the National Comorbidity Survey. Arch Gen Psychiatry 52:1048–1060, 1995

Kessler RC, Mroczek DK, Belli RF: Retrospective adult assessment of childhood psychopathology, in Assessment in Child and Adolescent Psychopathology. Edited by Shaffer D, Richters J. New York, Guilford (in press)

Kilpatrick DG, Resnick HS: Posttraumatic stress disorder associated with exposure to criminal victimization in clinical and community populations, in Posttraumatic Stress Disorder: DSM-IV and Beyond. Edited by Davidson JRT, Foa EB. Washington, DC, American Psychiatric Press, 1992, pp 113–143

Kilpatrick DG, Saunders BE, Veronen LJ, et al: Criminal victimization: lifetime prevalence, reporting to police, and psychological impact. Crime and Delinquency 33:479–489, 1987

Koopman C, Classen C, Spiegel D: Predictors of posttraumatic stress symptoms among survivors of the Oakland/Berkeley, Calif., firestorm. Am J Psychiatry 151:888–894, 1994

Koss MP: The scope of rape: implications for the clinical treatment of victims. Clinical Psychologist 36:88–91, 1983

Kulka RA, Schlenger WE, Fairbank JA, et al: Trauma and the Vietnam War Generation. New York, Brunner/Mazel, 1990

Lindemann E: Symptomatology and management of acute grief. Am J Psychiatry 101:141–148, 1944

March JS: What constitutes a stressor? The "Criterion A" issue, in Posttraumatic Stress Disorder: DSM-IV and Beyond. Edited by Davidson JRT, Foa EB. Washington, DC, American Psychiatric Press, 1992, pp 37–54

Martin E, Groves R, Mattlin J, et al: Report on Alternative Survey Procedures for the National Crime Survey. Washington, DC, Bureau of Social Science Research, 1986

Mellman TA, Randolph CA, Brawan-Mintzer O, et al: Phenomenology and course of psychiatric disorders associated with combat-related posttraumatic stress disorder. Am J Psychiatry 149:1568–1574, 1992

Parad H, Resnick H, Parad Z: Emergency Mental Health Services and Disaster Management. New York, Prentice-Hall, 1976

Perry S, Difede J, Musngi G, et al: Predictors of posttraumatic stress disorder after burn injury. Am J Psychiatry 149:931–935, 1992

Pynoos RS, Nader K: Children who witness the sexual assaults of their mothers. J Am Acad Child Adolesc Psychiatry 27:567–572, 1988

Resnick HS, Kilpatrick DG, Lipovsky JA: Assessment of rape-related posttraumatic stress disorder: stressor and symptom dimensions. J Consult Clin Psychol 3:561–572, 1991

Resnick HS, Kilpatrick DG, Dansky BS, et al: Prevalence of civilian trauma and posttraumatic stress disorder in a representative national sample of women. J Consult Clin Psychol 61:984–991, 1993

Robins LN, Wing J, Wittchen H-U, et al: The Composite International Diagnostic Interview: an epidemiologic instrument suitable for use in conjunction with different diagnostic systems and in different cultures. Arch Gen Psychiatry 45:1069–1077, 1988

Shore JH, Vollmer WM, Tatum EI: Community patterns of posttraumatic stress disorders. J Nerv Ment Dis 177:681–685, 1989

Sierles FS, Chen J, McFarland RE, et al: Posttraumatic stress disorder and concurrent psychiatric illness: a preliminary report. Am J Psychiatry 140:1177–1179, 1983

Solomon S, Canino G: Appropriateness of the DSM-III-R criteria for posttraumatic stress disorder. Compr Psychiatry 31:227–237, 1990

Solomon Z, Neria Y, Ohry A, et al: PTSD among Israeli former prisoners of war and soldiers with combat stress reaction: a longitudinal study. Am J Psychiatry 151:554–559, 1994

Spitzer RL, Williams JBW, Gibbon M, et al: Structured Clinical Interview for DSM-III-R—Patient Version (SCID-P). New York, New York State Psychiatric Institute, Biometrics Research, 1989

Warshaw MG, Fierman E, Pratt L, et al: Quality of life and dissociation in anxiety disorder patients with histories of trauma or PTSD. Am J Psychiatry 150:1512–1516, 1993

World Health Organization: Composite International Diagnostic Interview. Version 1.0. Geneva, World Health Organization, 1990a

World Health Organization: Composite International Diagnostic Interview [computer program]. Version 1.1. Geneva, World Health Organization, 1990b

World Health Organization: Composite International Diagnostic Interview. Version 2.1. Geneva, World Health Organization, 1997

Chapter 3

Genetic Risk Factors for PTSD: A Twin Study

William R. True, Ph.D., and Michael J. Lyons, Ph.D.

R esearch has indicated that there is a genetic influence on most human characteristics. It is misguided to ask whether a trait is determined either by genetic factors or by environmental factors. For virtually any trait of interest to psychologists and psychiatrists, both genetic and environmental influences are likely to be important. A better question is, What are the relative contributions of genetic and environmental factors, and how do each of these sets of factors operate?

It is particularly interesting to apply this question to posttraumatic stress disorder (PTSD) because, by definition, environmental determinants are a necessary factor in its etiology. Indeed,

This work was supported by the Department of Veterans Affairs Health Services Research and Development Service (Study 256). Partial support was provided by the National Institute on Drug Abuse (NIDA) (grant 1 R01 DAO 4604-01); the National Institute on Alcohol Abuse and Alcoholism (NIAAA grant 1 R01 AA10339-01); the Great Lakes Veterans Affairs Health Services Research and Development Program, Ann Arbor, MI (LIP 41-065); and the Public Health Service (grants MH-37685 and MH-31302). Work was also partially supported by NIDA training grant DAO72261–01 awarded to Washington University, St. Louis, MO.

The following organizations provided invaluable support in the conduct of this study: the staff of the Vietnam Era Twin Registry, Hines VA Medical Center, Hines, IL, Department of Defense; National Personnel Records Center, National Archives and Records Administration; Internal Revenue Service; National Opinion Research Center; National Research Council, National Academy of Sciences; and Institute for Survey Research, Temple University. We thank Jeffrey Scherrer, M.A., School of Public Health, St. Louis University Health Sciences Center, for his editorial work on this chapter. Most importantly, the authors gratefully acknowledge the continued cooperation and participation of the members of the Vietnam Era Twin Registry. Without their contribution this research would not have been possible.

PTSD may be seen as the quintessential environmentally determined psychopathology, since it is the only form of mental illness that requires the presence of an environmental risk factor (i.e., a traumatic event) as a criterion for the disorder. However, even when the environmental risk factors that are necessary for development of pathology have been identified, the possibility remains that genetic factors also contribute to liability for developing a disorder. For example, not all cigarette smokers develop lung cancer, even when the smokers under consideration use the same type and amount of tobacco. Similarly, not all individuals exposed to the same degree of trauma will develop symptoms of PTSD or the full-blown disorder.

Genetic Approaches to PTSD

Genetically informative designs for understanding the transmission of psychopathology include twin, family, and adoption studies. Family study designs have been applied to research in psychopathology such as depression, panic, and generalized anxiety (Davidson et al. 1989; McFarlane 1989; Reich et al. 1996), but full pedigrees have not been obtained for PTSD. Although potentially powerful tests of the heritability of psychopathology can be developed from adoption studies, the adoption method has not been applied in PTSD research. The lack of adoption studies of this disorder is not surprising considering the potential difficulties in identifying informative families.

Despite the limited information about the heritability of PTSD from family and adoption studies, resources for investigating genetic and environmental influences on PTSD are available in the Vietnam Era Twin Registry. A twin project is arguably the most informative experiment for understanding the genetics of PTSD, since the relative contributions of genes and environment can be assessed in a properly designed study. The present investigation is the first study of PTSD involving twins and the first to address directly the contribution of genetics to the etiology of PTSD with data collected from members of the Vietnam Era Twin Registry.

The feasibility of a twin design depends on the development of an adequately large population of identical and fraternal twins. In addition, a twin study of PTSD requires the identification of a sample of twins in which three combinations of traumatic exposure were applicable: 1) both members of a twin pair were exposed, 2) neither member of a pair was exposed, and 3) only one member of the pair was exposed. Obtaining such a sample was possible through the development of the Vietnam Era Twin Registry, a process begun in 1982 with initial exploration of administrative requirements and feasibility studies, culminating in the creation of a subject database and first survey of the registry members in 1987.

Vietnam Era Twin Registry

All registry members are males born between 1939 and 1957. To be eligible for membership, both brothers of the pair must have served in the military during the Vietnam War era, defined as 1965 to 1975. Twins were identified using archival computer tapes from the Department of Defense. It was necessary to develop a computerized algorithm to sort through approximately five million records from that time. With this algorithm, we identified pairs of individuals who had the same last name, different first names, and the same date of birth. We further verified that the members of a putative twin pair had similar social security numbers. Zygosity was determined by a questionnaire that included questions like "When you were little, did people often confuse you with your twin brother?" Questionnaire data were paired with military service blood group information for further verification. A description of this method for determining zygosity, about 95% accurate, has been published elsewhere (Eisen et al. 1989). Complete details regarding the construction of the Vietnam Era Twin Registry have been previously reported (Eisen et al. 1987; Henderson et al. 1990).

In 1987, all members of the Vietnam Era Twin Registry were invited to participate in the Survey of Health, which was intended to assess the physical and psychological effects of service in Vietnam. Special attention was given to adverse effects of chemical agent exposure, symptoms of posttraumatic stress, and exposure to wartime trauma. Registry members were sent a questionnaire, and those members who did not respond were contacted by phone. Response rates of 65% (pairwise) and 74.5% (casewise) were achieved. Reasons for nonresponse included refusal (9.5%), ineligibility (0.4%), death (2.7%), unavailability for study (i.e., either outside the United States or too ill to respond) (0.5%), and no response to repeated mailings or telephone calls (12.4%). Only pairs in which both members responded are informative for estimating the genetic and environmental contribution to PTSD.

Of the total Vietnam Era Twin Registry membership, 4,042 twin pairs met our inclusionary criteria and participated in the study. These consisted of 2,224 monozygotic (MZ) twin pairs and 1,818 dizygotic (DZ) twin pairs. The number of DZ twins in the general population is about double that of MZ twins, but the Vietnam Era Twin Registry consists of only male twin pairs, and therefore opposite-sex DZ twins could not be included. In addition, pairs of MZ twins tend to be more likely to participate in research than pairs of DZ twins, and this further increased the proportion of identical twin pairs.

Basic Characteristics of Twin Designs

Two sources of influence tend to make twins similar, and one source of influence tends to make them different. First, MZ twins, by definition, share all of their genes, whereas DZ twins share approximately half their genes, just as do any other siblings. Thus, MZ twins are twice as alike genetically as DZ twins. Further, both MZ and DZ twins have shared environmental experiences, seen particularly in the family rearing environment. Examples of shared environment include having parents who are both high school graduates; living in the same neighborhood; and going to the same schools. Genes and the shared or family environment, therefore, promote similarity within twin pairs. A third influence derives from unique environmental factors that contribute to dissimilarity within identical twin pairs. Unique environmental influences encompass a host of variables, measured and unmeasured, that one twin experienced but his brother did not. A pertinent example would be a twin pair in which one twin participated in military combat while his brother did not serve overseas.

Differences between DZ twins, as with MZ twins, are promoted by the unique environment as well as by the 50% of additive genetic influences that these twins do not share (i.e., there is a 50% chance of sharing one allele at a locus for additive genetic effects, and a 25% chance of sharing two alleles at the same locus in the case of dominant genetic effects). The basic univariate twin design is shown in Figure 3–1. A and D represent additive and dominant genetic influences, respectively, on the risk of developing PTSD. C represents shared environmental influences, and E represents

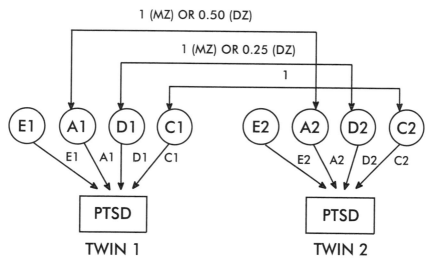

Figure 3–1. Basic genetic model (univariate twin design) for posttraumatic stress disorder (PTSD). A and D represent additive and dominant genetic influences, respectively, on the risk of developing PTSD. C represents shared environmental influences, and E represents unique environmental influences for PTSD. Additive genetic effects are those that increase the liability for expression of a phenotype in a linear fashion with each addition of an allele at a gene locus. Dominant genetic effects are those that nonadditively increase the expression of the trait. Either an additive (ACE) model or a nonadditive (ADE) model may be fit. MZ = monozygotic; DZ = dizygotic.

unique environmental influences for PTSD. Additive genetic effects are those that increase the liability for expression of a phenotype in a linear fashion with each addition of an allele at a gene locus. Dominant genetic effects are those that nonadditively increase the expression of the trait.

Application of the Twin Design Approach to PTSD

The 1987 Survey of Health contained a combat scale that assessed a range of combat experiences, including firing artillery, flying aircraft, serving as a "tunnel rat," and witnessing enemy or one's own casualties (Table 3–1). The validity of these self-reported combat experiences in relation to military records and decorations has been previously reported (Janes et al. 1991). A global combat index was developed by summing all positive responses from each subject. Scores were grouped into four approximate quartiles for military service: 1) non–Southeast Asia and Southeast Asia noncombat; 2) low combat; 3) medium combat; and 4) high combat. The test-retest reliability and validity of this scale have been previously reported (Janes et al. 1991; Lyons et al. 1993).

Table 3–1. Vietnam Era Twin Registry Survey of Health Combat Scale

1. In artillery unit: fired on enemy	10. Received incoming fire
2. Flew in aircraft	11. Encountered mines and booby traps
3. Flew attack gunships or medvacs	12. Received sniper fire
4. Stationed at a forward observation post	13. Unit patrol ambushed
5. Served as tunnel rat	14. Shot down while flying
6. Served on river patrol or gunboat	15. Engaged enemy in firefight
7. Demolitions expert in field	16. Saw soldiers killed
8. Retrieved dead/graves and registration	17. Was wounded
9. Served as medic in combat	18. Captured by the enemy

Source. Developed in collaboration with the late Robert S. Laufer.

The 1987 Survey of Health also collected data on PTSD-related symptoms through questions derived from the diagnostic criteria in DSM-III-R (American Psychiatric Association 1987). In DSM-III-R, PTSD symptoms are grouped into several symptom clusters: experiencing of a traumatic event outside the normal range of human experience (criterion A), reexperiencing of the trauma (criteria B), avoidance of stimuli associated with the trauma (criteria C), and persistent symptoms of increased arousal (criterion D).

The differences between a behavioral genetic approach and an epidemiological approach should be made clear for a full appreciation of the unique contributions of the former approach to understanding PTSD. The distinction between these two approaches stems, in part, from differences in the nature of the particular research question and the manner in which the data are organized and analyzed. The question from the epidemiological perspective is, What are the exposures that are associated with development of the disorder? The question from the genetic perspective is, What are the sources of variance contributing to susceptibility? Further comparison of the two approaches indicates how the genetic question follows logically from the epidemiological one.

Epidemiological Approach

Epidemiological approaches to PTSD typically use a cross-sectional design and examine prevalence rates. A classic study exemplifying this approach is that by Kessler and colleagues (1995). Studies using this approach have generally indicated that higher levels of trauma are associated with elevations in PTSD symptomatology. Data from one of our studies (True et al. 1993) can address this question. In Figure 3–2, the proportion of the study sample reporting reexperiencing symptoms (painful memories, nightmares, feelings as if events were happening again, and memories feeling stronger) is shown for four combat exposure levels. There is a monotonic relationship for each of the reexperiencing symptoms with the level of combat exposure. That relationship may be expressed in terms of a correlation coefficient—specifically,

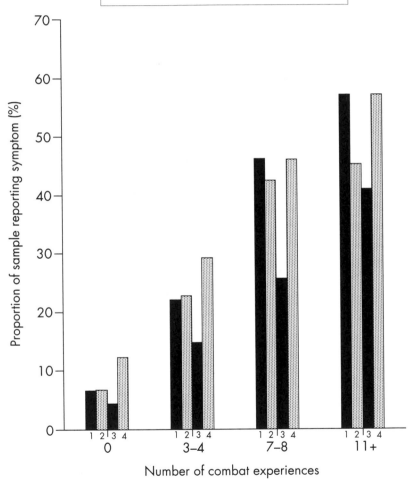

Figure 3–2. Association between posttraumatic stress disorder (PTSD) reexperiencing symptoms and level of combat exposure.
Source. Data from True et al. 1993.

a polychoric correlation (which is appropriate when both variables are ordinal). All of the correlations of reexperiencing symptoms with combat are substantial (i.e., 0.46 or higher). These data demonstrate a clear dose-response relationship between trauma and the intensity of reexperiencing symptoms.

The picture is more complex when the relationship between trauma and "avoidance" symptoms is examined (Figure 3–3). Only for "avoided activities" is there a very substantial correlation between combat exposure and the symptom. For the other PTSD symptoms, there is merely a modest correlation. Parallel data for increased arousal symptoms are presented in Figure 3–4. Note that the correlations are quite modest for the relationship between combat exposure and these PTSD symptoms.

Interestingly, as reported in other studies of Vietnam War veterans (Kulka et al. 1988; Wilson and Krauss 1985), there is a relationship between many PTSD symptoms and the level of combat exposure, but the relationship varies with the symptom cluster examined. Only for the "reexperiencing" cluster of symptoms is there a clear association with combat. A single symptom, "avoided activities," is the only avoidance symptom that is strongly correlated with combat, and all the increased arousal symptoms have very low correlations with combat. Therefore, combat, which is conventionally considered the primary etiological agent for PTSD, appears to be critical for only a subset of symptoms.

Behavioral Genetic Approach

We capitalized on the fact that our sample consisted of twins to take a step beyond the traditional epidemiological approach to include behavioral genetic techniques. About one-third of approximately 8,000 Vietnam Era Twin Registry respondents actually served in Vietnam. In the present study, we analyzed data from records of both those who served and those who did not serve in Vietnam. The question we addressed was, What are the genetic and environmental influences on susceptibility to PTSD? However, before we could accurately examine the individual susceptibility for PTSD symptoms, we had to account for familial

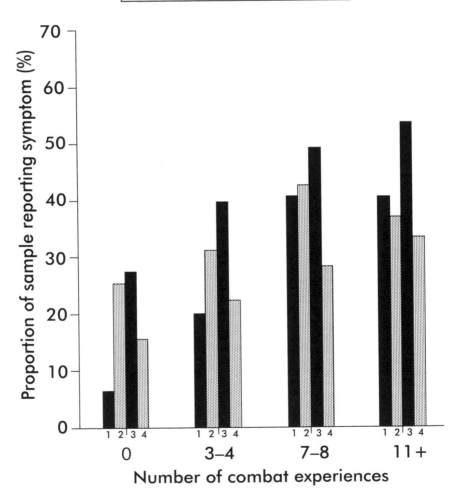

Figure 3–3. Association between posttraumatic stress disorder (PTSD) avoidance symptoms and level of combat exposure.
Source. Data from True et al. 1993.

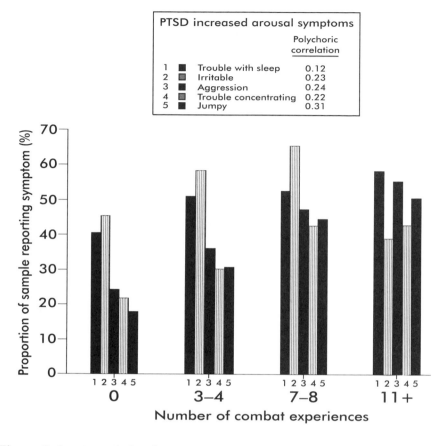

Figure 3–4. Association between posttraumatic stress disorder (PTSD) increased arousal symptoms and level of combat exposure.
Source. Data from True et al. 1993.

influences on DSM-III-R criterion A, exposure to "an event that is outside the range of usual human experience and that would be markedly distressing to almost anyone."

It may seem puzzling to suggest that the risk of experiencing a "random" traumatic event could be influenced by our genes and family environment. This assumption challenges the way we think of trauma. However, when we consider the possible role of personality factors such as risk taking or extroversion and introversion, it is plausible that some persons are more likely than others to experience events such as combat or physical assaults. Personality traits and other genetically influenced psychological characteristics may lead to some persons selecting themselves for risky behavior such as duty in frontline military units or demolition squads. Similarly, shared environmental experiences such as education, economic resources, and parental influences may affect the probability that an individual will join a branch of the military that is more likely to experience combat (i.e., service in frontline marine division vs. on a supply ship).

The Vietnam Era Twin Registry provided a unique opportunity for examining the relative genetic and environmental contributions to traumatic exposure, since data regarding volunteerism for service in Vietnam, exposure to a variety of combat situations, and military decorations are available from the 1987 Survey of Health. There were no restrictions on both twin members of a pair, one member of a pair, or neither twin serving in a particular branch of the military or field of operations. As with all other veterans, the members of the Vietnam Era Twin Registry could, to a degree, select themselves into or out of "risky" duty. Within the military, standardized tests, manpower requirements, and changing operations will reduce the individual soldier's ability to select the amount of risk in his environment. Thus, the twin structure allowed us to compute the heritability of exposing oneself to hazardous situations (e.g., volunteering for Vietnam service). We were also able to estimate the relative contribution of genes and shared environmental influences on combat trauma.

In this analysis, we focused on responses from 4,029 twin pairs to two questions—"While in the military did you request a Vietnam duty assignment?" and "When you were in the military, were you stationed in Vietnam, Laos, or Cambodia; in the waters in or around these countries; or fly in missions over these areas?"—and to the 18 combat-specific questions discussed earlier in this chapter. Based on these responses, we estimated the amount of variance due to genes and shared environmental influences on volunteering for service in Vietnam, combat exposure, and combat decorations.

Genetic factors accounted for 36% of the variance in Southeast Asia service, 47% of the variance in combat exposure, and 54% of the variance in likelihood of receiving a combat medal. Shared environmental factors did not significantly contribute to likelihood of any of these traumatic exposures.

It may be surprising to many that the early family rearing environment did not contribute to risk of wartime trauma. However, we believe that our results are consistent with a number of other findings. Other researchers have shown that personality characteristics such as sensation seeking, impulsivity, and extroversion are strongly influenced by additive genetic effects, with little or no shared environmental impact (Loehlin 1992). Since extroverted persons and sensation-seeking persons are more likely to experience traumatic events (Breslau et al. 1991; Mawson et al. 1988), possibly by seeking out stressors, individuals contribute to their own environments in part because of the genetic influence on their personality. Of course, sensation-seeking persons do not seek to develop PTSD or to experience trauma; however, when individuals repeatedly expose themselves to dangerous situations, they may cross an exposure threshold and come to represent an affected case.

Members of the Vietnam Era Twin Registry may have increased their liability for combat exposure through a number of mechanisms. Standardized tests were used to classify personnel to infantry duty, technical positions, or administrative roles. Volunteerism could have increased the likelihood of serving in a combat zone or in special forces. In one study, military personnel who volunteered for special forces helicopter training and those who completed more standard training were found to have different personality profiles (Caldwell et al. 1993); in this case, genetically influenced personality profiles influenced the amount of stress recruits were seeking, under the assumption that special forces training would result in more hazardous duty. We must also acknowledge that the impact of the environment could have been different if data were available from twins who did not serve in the military during the Vietnam War era. However, it is clear that trauma as required for a diagnosis of PTSD is not always a random event and is at least partially influenced by the individual. Clearly, some traumatic events are random or "fateful," but others may be associated with aspects of the individual that increase or decrease the risk of exposure.

Having established a genetic contribution to trauma, we then examined the risk for PTSD in a bivariate design that accounts for genes contributing to both PTSD and traumatic exposure. Using LISREL statistical software, we performed bivariate path analyses. A bivariate analysis, in terms of biometrical modeling, involves evaluation of two outcome variables simultaneously, in which their possible interrelationship is taken into account. In the present case, PTSD symptomatology and exposure to combat were examined at the same time. When we evaluated the determinants of variance in liability for PTSD, we included potential genetic and environmental factors that influence both the likelihood of being exposed to combat and the risk of traumatic stress symptomatology. (We might have reached a spurious conclusion about genetic influences on PTSD if we had not taken into account genetic influences common to combat exposure and PTSD.)

After performing the above analyses, we were able to examine the proportion of variance in risk for PTSD symptoms due to genes and environment (Figure 3–5). "Gn" refers to heritability, and "En" represents the environmental experiences unique to each member of a twin pair. Individual differences in having a "reexperiencing" symptom are partially the result of genetic factors. For the symptom "painful memories," only about 10% of the variance in liability for this symptom was found to be attributable to genes, but for the other "reexperiencing" symptoms, genes accounted for approximately 30% of the variance in risk. The remaining variance in risk for individual symptoms of PTSD was attributable to unique environmental experiences. To account for all unique experiences, we would need to have data on an infinite number of variables. However, because we adjusted for the effects of combat exposure, our estimate of the genetic and environmental contributions to these symptoms includes the effects of combat trauma. As with "reexperiencing symptoms," we found that genes accounted for approximately 30% of the risk for each symptom of "avoidance" and each symptom of "increased arousal." One exception was the relatively small influence from genes to liability for the symptom "trouble with sleep."

One conclusion from these bivariate analyses is that after genetic

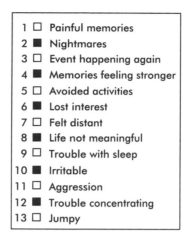

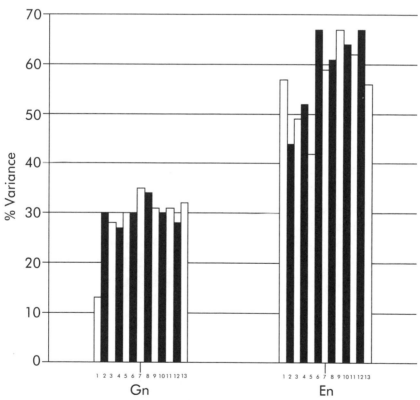

Figure 3–5. Variance in risk of posttraumatic stress disorder (PTSD) symptoms due to genes (Gn) and environment (En) after liability for combat exposure was controlled.
Source. Data from True et al. 1993.

influences on exposure to trauma are controlled, there is a significant genetic influence on susceptibility to PTSD. After combat exposure is taken into account, there is still a substantial genetic influence on how vulnerable an individual is to developing PTSD. Aspects of parental treatment applied similarly to both twins have no detectable influence on risk of developing PTSD given exposure to trauma, at least according to our data.

Conclusion

We have demonstrated a genetic influence on susceptibility to symptoms of PTSD that is partially shared with the risk for traumatic exposure. The impact of genetic vulnerability varies by symptom. For example, the risk of developing painful memories after a traumatic experience appears to be more a function of environmental influences, whereas symptoms of avoidance tend to be more genetically influenced. Although speculative, our data suggest that individuals may vary in their risk for different PTSD symptom profiles after traumatic exposure. We need to note that the relative magnitude of heritability observed in this study applies specifically to this population. The relative impact of genes and shared experiences may differ in females, in different age groups, and across cultures. The mechanisms of the genetic and the environmental influences are not specified in our results. We may expand our knowledge by identifying the mechanisms through which genes operate to increase susceptibility for PTSD symptoms. Future research should focus on how genetic factors influence biological substrates of this stress response.

References

American Psychiatric Association: Diagnostic and Statistical Manual of Mental Disorders, 3rd Edition, Revised. Washington, DC, American Psychiatric Association, 1987

Breslau N, Davis GC, Andreski P, et al: Traumatic events and posttraumatic stress disorder in an urban population of young adults. Arch Gen Psychiatry 48:216–222, 1991

Caldwell JA, O'Hara C, Caldwell JL, et al: Personality profiles of U.S. Army helicopter pilots screened for special operations duty. Military Psychology 5:187–199, 1993

Davidson J, Smith R, Kudler H: Familial psychiatric illness in chronic posttraumatic stress disorder. Compr Psychiatry 30:339–345, 1989

Eisen SA, True WR, Goldberg J, et al: The Vietnam Era Twin (VET) Registry: method of construction. Acta Genet Med Gemellol (Roma) 36:61–66, 1987

Eisen SA, Neuman R, Goldberg J, et al: Determining zygosity in the Vietnam Era Twin Registry: an approach using questionnaires. Clin Genet 35:423–432, 1989

Henderson WG, Eisen SA, Goldberg J, et al: The Vietnam Era Twin Registry: a resource for medical research. Public Health Rep 105:368–373, 1990

Janes GR, Goldberg J, Eisen SA, et al: Reliability and validity of a combat exposure index for Vietnam era veterans. J Clin Psychol 47:80–86, 1991

Kessler RC, Sonnega A, Bromet W, et al: Posttraumatic stress disorder in the National Comorbidity Survey. Arch Gen Psychiatry 52:1048–1060, 1995

Kulka RA, Schlenger WE, Fairbank JA, et al: Contractual Report of Findings From the National Vietnam Veterans Readjustment Study. Research Triangle Park, NC, Research Triangle Institute, 1988

Loehlin JC: Genes and Environment in Personality Development. Newbury Park, CA, Sage, 1992

Lyons MJ, Goldberg J, Eisen SA, et al: Do genes influence exposure to trauma? A twin study of combat. Am J Med Genet (Neuropsychiatric Genetics) 48:22–27, 1993

Mawson AR, Jacobs KW, Winchester Y, et al: Sensation-seeking and traumatic spinal cord injury: case-control study. Arch Phys Med Rehabil 69:1039–1043, 1988

McFarlane AC: The aetiology of post-traumatic morbidity: predisposing, precipitating and perpetuating factors. Br J Psychiatry 154:221–228, 1989

Reich J, Lyons M, Cai B: Familial vulnerability factors to post-traumatic stress disorder in male military veterans. Acta Psychiatr Scand 93: 105–112, 1996

True WR, Rice J, Eisen SA, et al: A twin study of genetic and environmental contributions to liability for posttraumatic stress symptoms. Arch Gen Psychiatry 50:257–264, 1993

Wilson JP, Krauss GE: Predicting post-traumatic stress disorders among Vietnam veterans, in Post-Traumatic Stress Disorder and the War Veteran Patient. Edited by Kelly WE. New York, Brunner/Mazel, 1985, pp 102–147

Chapter 4

Family Studies of PTSD: A Review

Jonathan R. T. Davidson, M.D., and
Kathryn M. Connor, M.D.

During the first World War of 1914 to 1918, psychiatric attention was concentrated on the clinical manifestations of neurosis ("shell shock") and on its psychological causes. During the second World War, attention was given more to the constitutional background. It was found that the liability to neurotic breakdown varied with the degree of stress imposed, but also with the degree of constitutional instability. This constitutional factor could be detected and to some extent measured by . . . a family history of nervous illness, a past history of nervous breakdown or an irregular work record.

The constitutional liability to neurosis varied quantitatively but was not of a unitary kind. Some men were highly susceptible to stress of one kind, others to another. . . . the nature of the symptoms, however, was found to have close associations with the basic personality of the patient, and somewhat less close ones with the type of stress to which he had been subjected. Certain types of environment had a preferential effect in producing anxiety symptoms, others . . . depression, others . . . hypochondriacal preoccupation. In general, however, forms frustes of the eventually incapacitating neurotic symptoms could be found in the patient's past life, and were associated with the makeup of his personality. (Slater and Roth 1972, pp 61–62)

This passage from Slater and Roth's (1972) book penetrates to a critical, and yet poorly understood, determinant of posttraumatic stress disorder (PTSD), namely, the constitutional-hereditary factor. While we have substantially advanced our knowledge of the causes of PTSD since the above comments were made, this description from an earlier generation still captures an important part of our current understanding about the complex etiology of PTSD. Slater and Roth also pointed out that at different times in its development, psychiatry has shifted its focus from one area (e.g., symptoms or psychological causes) to another (e.g., constitution or biological factors). The authors also acknowledged the interactive, and probably reciprocal, relationship between predisposition and severity of stress and raised the intriguing possibility that type of stressor is related to the development of particular symptoms, a relationship that makes even more difficult the business of disentangling hereditary predisposition for PTSD. (Authors of subsequent work [e.g., Laufer et al. 1985; Solomon and Canino 1990] also have observed a determining effect of environmental stress on the particular symptom picture that results.) Finally, Slater and Roth recognized that pure forms of stress-induced disorder are relatively rare and that in the majority of neurotic patients anxiety and hysterical symptoms are found together.

Notwithstanding the numerous challenges facing us, some degree of uniformity has emerged from the many family investigations conducted with respect to PTSD. Nonetheless, there remain a number of inconsistencies that force us to think carefully about the essence of PTSD, an already complex pattern reflective of more than one pathogenic process. Furthermore, an investigation of risk factors for PTSD requires that we distinguish between risk for developing symptoms and risk for exposure to trauma.

The importance of heredity as a determinant of psychiatric disorders is well established for a variety of conditions, including schizophrenia, major depression, bipolar disorder, anxiety disorders, personality disorders, and alcoholism. In and of itself, a positive family history does not indicate to us whether the illness is determined through genetic mechanisms, environmental factors, or a combination of both. However, the existence of familial transmission in a disease is considered to be one traditional way of validating a disease entity and may help us further understand its mechanism (Robins and Guze 1970).

In this chapter, we describe the literature on familial pathology among individuals identified as experiencing PTSD or historically related syndromes. A recent study of rape victims is also briefly described. We then outline methodological considerations in family studies of PTSD and consider their implications for future studies.

Familial Psychopathology and Stress-Induced Syndromes

One of the earliest references to inherited predisposition was the report on a group of World War I combat veterans by Wolfsohn (1918), who conducted a controlled study involving 100 patients with war neurosis and 100 matched control subjects with war-related physical injuries. Wolfsohn found that 74% of the war neurosis patients in his sample reported a family history of "psychoneurosis," which covered a broad spectrum of conditions, including nervousness, alcoholism, epilepsy, and insanity. No positive family history of such disorders was reported by any of the control subjects. Although the possibility of interview bias cannot be excluded, the study used a carefully matched design.

In 1918 two other reports—those by Oppenheimer and Rothschild (1918) and Robey and Boaz (1918)—evaluated British and American World War I combatants. In the study of British soldiers (Oppenheimer and Rothschild 1918), 56% of subjects with "shell shock" reported a family history of psychoneurosis, which, as in Wolfsohn's study, included nervousness, alcoholism, irascibility, insanity, and epilepsy. In the U.S. study (Robey and Boaz 1918), the great majority of 89 hospitalized patients reported a family history of "nervous disorder," with first-degree relatives often tending to be nervous, irritable, and easily upset.

Shortly after the end of World War I, Swan (1921) found that of 58 U.S. returnees who had been evaluated and found to have shell shock, 52% reported a family history of nervous disease, including insanity, suicide, syphilis, alcoholism, and depression.

Thus, the World War I studies consistently found a high rate (52% to 74%) of a wide variety of familial psychopathology, with the emphasis on predominantly the extent of nervousness and irritability.

Several family investigations were conducted with World War II soldiers with war neurosis (Cohen et al. 1948; Curran and Mallinson 1940). Curran and Mallinson (1940) compared family histories of 100 British returnees with war neurosis with those of 50 surgical control subjects. Forty-five percent of the soldiers with war neurosis had a positive family history as defined by a parent, aunt, or sibling's either having been in a mental hospital or attempted suicide or having shown evidence of functionally impairing psychiatric illness that did not result in hospitalization. Despite adopting quite stringent criteria for defining a case, the investigators in this study still found a relatively high rate of psychopathology (45%) among families of the affected soldiers.

Cohen and colleagues (1948) compared family histories of 144 U.S. World War II service personnel with neurocirculatory asthenia (NCA) with those of 105 healthy control subjects and another control group of 48 veterans and medical patients. A history of NCA was noted in 58% of mothers, 18.5% of fathers, and 12.6% of siblings in the NCA group. No such histories were noted in the control groups. Cohen et al. also interviewed 15 family members of the NCA group and corroborated the history in all cases. This study represents the first attempt at a direct family interview among patients with PTSD-related disorders. Although NCA does not correspond exactly with the criteria for PTSD, there is substantial overlap, and it is not unreasonable to consider these findings as being relevant to the study of PTSD.

In a subsequent study of World War II veterans, evaluated several decades after the termination of conflict, and a group of Vietnam veterans, Davidson and colleagues (1985) found high rates of familial psychopathology (66%), with alcoholism, depression, and anxiety being noted most often. In another study conducted long after the end of World War II, Speed and colleagues (1989) noted that family history of mental illness, including alcoholism, was weakly correlated with persistent PTSD symptoms in World War II POWs. In Speed et al.'s judgment, the severity of the trauma takes precedence over familial factors in terms of their role in the development of PTSD. These findings raise the possibility that under the most extreme forms of stress and deprivation, inherited predisposition is outweighed by the enormity of the stressor. In other words, more resilient individuals require higher levels of stress to evoke PTSD, as noted by Slater (1943).

Civilian studies over the last 50 years have demonstrated similar findings of familiality. In a study of civilians with NCA, Wheeler and colleagues (1948) observed that 48.6% of these civilians' offspring, as compared with 5.6% of control probands' offspring, reported NCA. In a more recent study, McFarlane (1988) found a family history of unspecified psychiatric illness in 55% of volunteer firefighters who had been exposed to severe fires and developed PTSD, as compared with 20% in volunteers without PTSD.

Epidemiological investigations of PTSD have also provided evidence of heritability. In a report from the Epidemiologic Catchment Area (ECA) study conducted in North Carolina, Davidson and colleagues (1991) noted that respondents with PTSD were three times more likely to report family mental illness than were control subjects. The authors noted no increase in familial alcoholism, however. In another U.S. epidemiological study, conducted in Detroit, Breslau and colleagues (1991) observed an increase in family rates of anxiety, depression, psychosis, and antisocial behavior. As with the ECA study, no increase was found for family alcoholism, and this suggests that raised rates may be confined to combat trauma populations. In this respect, it is also possible that men and women with PTSD exhibit different patterns of family psychopathology.

The possibility of gender-related differences in the genetics of PTSD and other disorders has been raised by Krystal and colleagues (1996) and by Kosten and co-workers (1991). Clearly, it is necessary to undertake multiple types of family investigation in PTSD that take into account an adequate sample of men and women, as well as to control for type of trauma (e.g., military combat, sexual trauma, accidental injury, natural disaster). In addition, a standardized form of measurement for trauma severity would be useful given the considerations raised above regarding the reciprocal relationship between trauma intensity and individual vulnerability. To date, trauma severity scales have focused on particular events (e.g., combat, rape).

Only one family study of PTSD has so far been conducted. In this study, which assessed family psychopathology as a possible risk factor for chronic PTSD (i.e., duration of more than 6 months) after rape, Davidson and colleagues (unpublished data) found that depression was increased in first-degree relatives of probands with PTSD compared with healthy control subjects, and anxiety was only weakly so. Rates of alcohol or substance use disorder were not increased. Rates of alcohol use disorder in the relatives of rape trauma victims with and without PTSD and in healthy control subjects were 12.6%, 8.2%, and 6.3%, respectively. Rates of drug use disorder in the three groups were 4.4%, 3.1%, and 1.9%. Again, these results do not suggest a link between PTSD and substance use disorders among civilians, but they do point to a tie between PTSD and depression in a rape-related PTSD population.

An innovative approach has been used by Nagy and colleagues (Nagy 1993) that investigates the relation of biological abnormality to family history. In their study of Vietnam War veterans with PTSD, these authors found that yohimbine-induced panic attacks were not a marker of family-based panic disorder, because the rates of panic disorder among first-degree relatives of PTSD probands were not increased. Studies of this kind may prove to be immensely useful in helping us to better understand the biology of and risk factors for PTSD.

Methodological Considerations

Studies of familial psychopathology have demonstrated positive risk factors for alcoholism (Pitts and Winokur 1966), affective disorder (Coryell et al. 1984; Kupfer et al. 1989; Weissman et al. 1984), schizophrenia (Kendler et al. 1985), generalized anxiety disorder (Skre et al. 1993), social phobia (Fyer et al. 1993), panic disorder/agoraphobia (Noyes et al. 1987; Skre et al. 1993), obsessive-compulsive disorder (Pauls et al. 1995), and simple phobia (Fyer et al. 1990).

Typically, information about family psychiatric illness is obtained either through a family history from the proband or other relative covering all known family members or directly through an interview with the relative. The family history technique is simple, efficient, and economical. The specificity is high (i.e., a positive diagnosis is generally an accurate one), but the sensitivity is low (i.e., numerous actual cases of a disorder are missed) (Andreasen et al. 1977; Heun et al. 1982; Mendlewicz et al. 1975; Thompson et al. 1982). In a study by Heun and colleagues (1982), which looked at family history of dementia, the specificity for depression and/or dementia was more than 95%, but the sensitivity ranged from 10% to 40%. They noted that relatives of patients were better informants than relatives of control subjects for the presence of any psychiatric disorder. They also observed that the use of several informants only slightly improved the sensitivity of the family history and did not reduce the specificity, a finding that raises questions about the utility of involving several informants for a family history study. Family history assessment of anxiety disorders in particular may lack sensitivity, since the external markers are less obvious than would be the case for, say, serious depression, schizophrenia, or alcohol-related problems.

The family study method is more costly and time consuming but does produce somewhat more accurate data with higher rates of sensitivity. Data obtained by direct face-to-face interview or on the telephone appear to be equally as acceptable and valid (Abrams and Taylor 1983; Sobin et al. 1993).

Family history data are prone to recall bias, since not all psychiatric disorders will be observed and reported by family members. Family study information can also be influenced by selection bias, and in the case of PTSD it is questionable how accurate some of the data would be when PTSD is related to a dysfunctional family environment where, for example, abuse and incest have taken place. This level of potential inaccuracy makes difficult indeed the likelihood of applying the family study method to a fully representative spectrum of the PTSD population. Moreover, the genetics and family risk factors of PTSD arising in childhood in the context of a dysfunctional family may well differ from those related to PTSD that develops in a previously stable adult after a serious accident. Studies of combat veterans have been limited to males for the most part, whereas those in the community have included males and females. A family study of rape survivors (Davidson et al., unpublished data) was limited to females. Another important group, displaced persons and refugees with PTSD, would also be difficult to evaluate by means of the family study method. Nevertheless, a broad base drawn from men and women exposed to a variety of traumas is still needed for a more complete picture of family risks in relation to PTSD.

Conclusion

Numerous factors must be considered in furthering our understanding of inherited risk factors for PTSD (Table 4–1). These include consideration of gender, type of trauma, severity of trauma, and vulnerability to other, non-PTSD syndromes. Different methodologies of investigation should be brought to bear, including family history, direct interview, twin studies, and genetic marker studies, the last-mentioned of which has not yet been undertaken to our knowledge. Two twin studies have supported, respectively, heritability for most PTSD symptoms in U.S. Vietnam veterans (True et al. 1993) and the diagnosis of PTSD in Scandinavian anxiety disorder patients (Skre et al. 1993).

Family history studies of combat veterans seem to be fairly consistent in indicating heightened vulnerability in terms of anxiety, depressive, "neurotic," and/or alcohol or substance use problems.

Table 4–1.   Important methodological considerations for family risk studies of PTSD

---

1. Are family patterns of psychiatric disorder the same for men and women with PTSD?

2. Are findings invariant for type of trauma?

3. Were relatives interviewed directly?

4. Has the risk of trauma exposure in relatives been separated from risk of PTSD?

5. Has proband comorbidity been taken into account in evaluating results?

Furthermore, studies of World War II and Vietnam War veterans point to the reciprocal relationship between severity of trauma and predisposition for psychopathology. Civilian studies, although indicating familial psychopathology to be a risk factor, suggest that rates of family alcohol/substance abuse problems are not elevated in probands with PTSD. Also, the results from these studies regarding the relationship of PTSD and vulnerability to anxiety per se are mixed. To the extent that studies have not shown such a relationship, the rationale for the existing classification of PTSD as an anxiety disorder is weakened. Our family study of rape trauma victims suggests that depressive vulnerability is more important than anxiety as a risk factor for PTSD. Moreover, a multivariate regression of the data from this study, in which preexisting vulnerability to depression was included along with other risk factors (e.g., trauma severity, perceived life threat, age at trauma), indicated that preexisting vulnerability to depression remained an independent risk factor.

Another interesting strategy that could be adopted in future studies would be to consider not so much PTSD as a diagnosis, but vulnerability to some of the specific aspects of PTSD. For example, startle proneness may be related to alterations in chromosome number 5 (Ryan et al. 1992), can be familial, and may be related to a defect in the regulation of GABA, an inhibitory neurotransmitter (Dubowitz et al. 1992). Another component of PTSD in some cases, proneness to violent behavior, may be related to an impairment in serotonin synthesis resulting from genetic abnormality (Krystal et al. 1996). Behavioral inhibition/timidity in children is also related to genetic predisposition (Kagan et al. 1988).

PTSD is defined as a complex of different pathogenic characteristics. Thus, in some individuals, the salient clinical picture may be of depression, guilt, withdrawal, and numbing; in others, it may take the form of hyperarousal, startle, and hypervigilance; and in yet others, it may be characterized by swings of impulsivity, violence, and alcohol abuse. To what extent these presentations reflect a common underlying vulnerability versus manifestations of different vulnerabilities, all having one factor in common, namely, exposure to extreme stress, is still very much a question for debate.

Our study of family risk factors among rape victims points to the importance of comorbidity in PTSD, with PTSD comorbid for depression and PTSD in the absence of depression associated with different familial patterns of psychiatric disorder.

In 1919, Mott observed that there may be different vulnerabilities behind the development of PTSD. He stated that

> a large minority of shell-shock cases occur in persons with a nervous temperament, or persons who were the victims of an acquired, or inherited, neuropathy; also a neuro-potentially sound soldier in this trench warfare may, from stress of a prolonged active service, acquire a neurasthenic condition. If in a soldier there is an inborn timidity or neuropathic disposition, or an inborn germinal of acquired neuropathic or psychopathic taint causing a *locus minoris resistentia*, it necessarily follows that he will be less able to withstand the terrifying effects of shell fire and the stress of trench warfare. (Wolfson 1918)

Whether vulnerability to PTSD is related to predisposition to a particular disease, to neuroticism in general, or to some other factor has yet to be determined.

In summary, the field is at an exciting point, where the task is still to try to define better what questions need to be asked in order to help us further understand the vulnerability factors that predispose an individual to developing PTSD.

References

Abrams R, Taylor MA: The genetics of schizophrenia: a reassessment using modern research criteria. Am J Psychiatry 140:171–175, 1983

Andreasen NC, Endicott J, Spitzer RL, et al: The family history method using diagnostic criteria: reliability and validity. Arch Gen Psychiatry 34:1229–1235, 1977

Cohen ME, White PD, Johnson RE: Neurocirculatory asthenia, anxiety neurosis or the effort syndrome. Arch Intern Med 81:260–281, 1948

Coryell W, Endicott J, Reich T, et al: A family study of Bipolar II Disorder. Br J Psychiatry 145:49–54, 1984

Curran D, Mallinson WP: War-time psychiatry and economy in manpower. Lancet 2:738–743, 1940

Davidson JRT, Swartz M, Storck M, et al: A diagnostic and family study of posttraumatic stress disorder. Am J Psychiatry 142:90–93. 1985

Davidson JR, Hughes D, Blazer D, et al: Posttraumatic stress disorder in the community: an epidemiological study. Psychol Med 21:713–721, 1991

Dubowitz LMS, Bouz AH, Hird MF, et al: Low cerebrospinal fluid concentration of free gamma-aminobutyric acid in startle disease. Lancet 340:80–81, 1992

Fyer AJ, Mannuzza S, Gallops MS, et al: Familial transmission of simple phobias and fears. Arch Gen Psychiatry 47:252–256, 1990

Fyer AJ, Mannuzza S, Chapman TF, et al: A direct interview family study of social phobia. Arch Gen Psychiatry 50:286–293, 1993

Heun R, Hardt J, Burkhart M, et al: Validity of the family history method in relatives of gerontopsychiatric patients. Psychiatry Res 62:227–238, 1982

Kagan J, Reznick JS, Snidman N: Biological basis of childhood shyness. Science 240:167–171, 1988

Kendler KS, Gruenberg AM, Tsuang MT: Psychiatric illness in first-degree relatives of schizophrenic and surgical control patients: a family study using DSM-III criteria. Arch Gen Psychiatry 42:770–779, 1985

Kosten TR, Rounsaville BJ, Kosten TA, et al: Gender differences in the specificity of alcoholism transmission among the relatives of opioid addicts. J Nerv Ment Dis 179:392–400, 1991

Krystal JH, Nagy LM, Rasmussen A, et al: Initial clinical evidence of genetic contributions to post-traumatic stress disorder, in An International Handbook of Multigenerational Legacies of Trauma. Edited by Danieli Y. New York, Plenum, 1996, pp 657–667

Kupfer DJ, Frank E, Carpenter LL, et al: Family history in recurrent depression. J Affect Disord 17:113–119, 1989

Laufer RS, Frey-Woulters E, Gallops MS: Traumatic stressors in Vietnam veterans and post-traumatic stress disorder, in Trauma and Its Wake: The Study of Treatment of Post-Traumatic Stress Disorders. Edited by Figley CR. New York, Brunner-Mazel, 1985, pp 73–89

McFarlane AC: The aetiology of post-traumatic stress disorders following a natural disaster. Br J Psychiatry 152:116–121, 1988

Mendlewicz J, Fleiss JL, Cataldo M, et al: Accuracy of the family history method in affective illness: comparison with direct interviews in family studies. Arch Gen Psychiatry 32:309–314, 1975

Mott FW: War Neuroses and Shell Shock. London, Oxford Medical Publications, 1919

Nagy LM: Genetic study of PTSD: a family history study. Presentation at the annual meeting of the International Society of Traumatic Stress Studies, San Antonio, TX, October 1993

Noyes R, Clarkson CC, Crowe RR, et al: A family study of generalized anxiety disorder. Am J Psychiatry 144:1019–1024, 1987

Oppenheimer BS, Rothschild MA: The psychoneurotic factor in the irritable heart of soldiers. JAMA 70:1919–1922, 1918

Pauls DL, Alsobrook JP, Goodman W, et al: A family study of obsessive-compulsive disorder. Am J Psychiatry 152:76–84, 1995

Pitts FN, Winokur G: Affective disorder, VII: alcoholism and affective disorder. J Psychiatr Res 4:37–50, 1966

Robey WH, Boaz EP: Neurocirculatory asthenia. JAMA 71:525–529, 1918

Robins E, Guze SB: Establishment of diagnostic validity in psychiatric illness: its application to schizophrenia. Am J Psychiatry 126:107–111, 1970

Ryan SG, Sherman SL, Terry JC, et al: Startle disease or hyperekplexia: response to clonazepam and assignment of the gene (STHE) to chromosome 5 q linkage analysis. Ann Neurol 31:663–668, 1992

Skre I, Onstad S, Torgersen S, et al: A twin study of DSM-III-R anxiety disorders. Acta Psychiatr Scand 88:85–92, 1993

Slater E: The neurotic constitution: a statistical study of two thousand neurotic soldiers. Journal of Neurology and Psychiatry 6:1–16, 1943

Slater EO, Roth M: Clinical Psychiatry. London, Bailliere, Tyndall & Cassell, 1972

Sobin C, Weissman MM, Goldstein RB, et al: Diagnostic interviewing for family studies: comparing telephone and face-to-face methods for the diagnosis of lifetime psychiatric disorders. Psychiatr Genet 3:227–233, 1993

Solomon SD, Canino CJ: Appropriateness of DSM-III-R criteria for post-traumatic stress disorder. Compr Psychiatry 31:227–237, 1990

Speed N, Engdahl B, Schwartz J, et al: Posttraumatic stress disorder as a consequence of the POW experience. J Nerv Ment Dis 177:147–153, 1989

Swan JM: An analysis of ninety cases of functional disease in soldiers. Arch Intern Med 28:586–602, 1921

Thompson WD, Orvaschel H, Prusoff BA, et al: An evaluation of the family history method for ascertaining psychiatric disorders. Arch Gen Psychiatry 39:53–58, 1982

True WR, Rice J, Eisen SA, et al: A twin study of genetic and environmental contributions to liability for posttraumatic stress symptoms. Arch Gen Psychiatry 50:257–264, 1993

Weissman MM, Gershon ES, Kidd KK, et al: Psychiatric disorders in the relatives of probands with affective disorders: the Yale University–National Institute of Mental Health Collaborative Study. Arch Gen Psychiatry 41:13–21, 1984

Wheeler EO, White PD, Reed E, et al: Familial incidence of neurocirculatory asthenia ("Anxiety Neurosis Effort Syndrome"). Presentation at the 40th annual meeting of the American Society for Clinical Investigation, Atlantic City, NJ, 1948

Wolfsohn JM: The predisposing factors of war psycho-neuroses. Lancet 1:177–180, 1918

Chapter 5

Parental PTSD as a Risk Factor for PTSD

Rachel Yehuda, Ph.D.

In the previous two chapters, the authors considered approaches for examining familial contributions to posttraumatic stress disorder (PTSD). Both chapters demonstrated that there is an increased risk for the development of PTSD among individuals who have a family member with either PTSD or a mood or anxiety disorder. True and Lyons, in Chapter 3, showed that there was a greater prevalence of PTSD among trauma survivors who had a twin with PTSD. The risk was greater for monozygotic twins than for dizygotic twins. Davidson and Connor, in Chapter 4, demonstrated that the parents and first-degree relatives of trauma survivors with PTSD had a greater prevalence of mood, anxiety, and substance use disorders compared with trauma survivors who did not develop PTSD.

Our research group at the Mount Sinai School of Medicine and the Bronx Veterans Affairs Hospital has taken an analogous ap-

---

The work summarized in this chapter was performed by an interdisciplinary team of clinical researchers over a period of 6 years. The diagnostic evaluations were performed by Drs. Karen Binder-Brynes, Milton Wainberg, Dan Aferiot, Ann Steiner, Steven Southwick, Alan Lehman, Earl Giller, Jr., Boaz Kahana, Abbie Elkin, and Tamar Duvdevani. The clinical staff of the Specialized Treatment Program for Holocaust Survivors (Drs. Edith Laufer, Sheila Erlich, Jutta Weiss, Ruth Heber, Morton Seigel, Robert Grossman, Elizabeth Ronis, Burt Rosen, and Ilana Breslau) have been a wonderful source of wisdom regarding intergenerational issues. Also acknowledged are the wonderful administrative assistance and data management skills of Skye Wilson, Abbie Elkin, Stacey Namm, and Tamar Duvdevani. Cortisol determinations were performed by Drs. Kwei Yang and Ling Song Guo. We thank Shelley Zemelman for helping recruit the subjects from Cleveland, Ohio, and Dr. James Schmeidler for statistical consultation. This work was supported by grants from the National Institute of Mental Health (R01–49555 and R02-49555) to Dr. Yehuda.

proach to the study of risk, in that we have been particularly interested in exploring PTSD in first-degree relatives of trauma
survivors. However, rather than focusing on siblings or parents,
we have been interested in the adult children of trauma survivors.
In addition to examining life history and psychiatric diagnoses in
these first-degree relatives, our work has also included an assessment of neuroendocrine measures in trauma-surviving parents
and their children. This chapter summarizes our findings.

Evolution of the Present Research Studies on Offspring of Holocaust Survivors

When we began our studies of adult offspring of trauma survivors,
we did not know that we would ultimately be studying risk for
PTSD. That our results might be relevant to risk for PTSD is a post
hoc conclusion based on the findings of an increased prevalence of
this disorder in adult offspring, as summarized in what follows.

Our work began in response to what we perceived was a clinical
challenge and need. Our research group had for several years been
studying the neuroendocrinology of PTSD in different groups of
trauma survivors. Several years ago we began to study Holocaust
survivors. In addition to establishing a research program, we
opened a clinic in order to meet the treatment needs of aging Holocaust survivors. As our program became known in the New York
metropolitan community, we increasingly found that it was the
children of Holocaust survivors who called and asked to be treated
and studied. We responded to the request of these offspring and
opened up a program for the evaluation and treatment of children
of Holocaust survivors.

At first we simply listened informally to what these adult children had to say both in individual sessions and in our short-term
psychotherapy groups. It became clear to us very quickly that for
many offspring, having a Holocaust survivor parent had deeply affected them. What the Holocaust offspring expressed to us was
that as they became adults, and as they mentally compared themselves with others (i.e., individuals similar to them except for the
fact that their parents were not Holocaust survivors), they felt dif-

ferent and in some ways even "damaged." Some were able to articulate their feelings in more detail than others, but even the best descriptions of "damage" reflected a sense of vagueness about the nature and etiology of what they were experiencing.

Almost all children of Holocaust survivors told us that they felt like casualties of the Holocaust just like their parents. Some offspring told us that the actual stories they heard from their parents about their Holocaust experiences were extremely distressing to them. Some were too young to hear details of such graphic violence and were frightened as parents, often becoming quite emotional, relived these experiences. Some spoke about the physical and emotional damage to their parents and how this often resulted in an emotional and/or physical neglect of the child (i.e., the offspring). In some cases, we heard about acts of physical violence and sexual abuse by parents toward their children. Some offspring told us that they had been terribly affected by the responsibility of caring for their disabled parent(s) from a young age. Many children spoke of how their parents minimized their children's life experiences as trivial in comparison to what they had experienced during the Holocaust and accused their children of failing to acknowledge the sacrifices they had made on the children's behalf.

Some offspring told us that they recognized how much their parents had tried to bring them up with love and attention and to put the past behind them. But even in such families where parents tried hard to conquer their past memories, offspring often felt the burden of compensating the parent for past losses. In these homes, offspring also felt an underlying lesson being taught to them about how dangerous the world really is and how everything they would come to take for granted could be snatched away in an instant, without warning, and with no recourse. Many offspring told us that, even as adults, they feared the environment as much as their parents did and continued to react to it with inappropriate hypervigilance and distrust—almost as if they were living in a world of Nazis or would-be Nazis. They described how feelings of fear and distrust of self and others extended to the most intimate interpersonal relationships, making true closeness with others challenging.

The paradox that was expressed to us was that many offspring felt traumatized even though they did not feel that they had undergone any "trauma." Although they could express their symptoms, they minimized their actual experiences. Perhaps, as one offspring suggested, whatever they went through could never be as bad as the Holocaust. Many offspring felt that they should feel grateful and lucky to be living after the Holocaust and not during it. Yet, rather than feeling lucky, they expressed sadness, anxiety, and despair.

We felt it a great challenge to respond to the implicit—sometimes explicit—question of these adult children of Holocaust survivors: What, indeed, was wrong with adult offspring of Holocaust survivors who presented to our clinic for treatment, and why were they so symptomatic? Among our clinical and research team we also wondered how generalizable these symptoms would be to all children of trauma survivors. After all, it was clear that the individuals choosing to speak to us were a self-selected group who were motivated by their desire and need to receive clinical treatment or tell their story.

In consulting the literature on the effects of trauma on the children of trauma survivors, we found that many of the statements that we had heard had already been documented in the form of clinical anecdotes and descriptions. We studied the literature carefully to help us form a model that would explain what appeared to be a universal—or at least typical—response of children of trauma survivors. After clarifying ideas about what some began to call the "intergenerational" effects of trauma, it was our intention to then apply some of the methodologies that we had developed in the study of trauma survivors to further elucidate the nature and, possibly, etiology of clinical symptoms in this group.

Literature Review

An extensive review indicated that, with few exceptions, the literature on adult offspring of Holocaust survivors was divided. On the one hand were descriptions of the adverse effects of the Holocaust on the second generation, and on the other, failures to find adverse effects of the Holocaust on offspring. Very few authors wrote about clinical heterogeneity among children of survivors, but in this regard the insightful observations of Danieli (1982) and Novac (1993) must be mentioned.

Generally, the observations that children of Holocaust survivors displayed an increased incidence of psychological problems (Barocas and Barocas 1983; Danieli 1981; Rakoff 1966; Rakoff et al. 1976; Trossman 1968) appeared first. The earliest observations were made while offspring were still young children and adolescents. Several groups of authors reported an unusually high incidence of depression, anxiety, and maladaptive behavior, such as conduct disorder, personality problems, inadequate maturity, excessive dependence, and poor coping problems, in these children (Rackoff et al. 1976). It was later observed that adult offspring of Holocaust survivors had more physical ailments (Waldfogel 1991) and psychological problems (Danieli 1981; Kestenberg 1972, 1980; Kinsler 1981; Last and Klein 1981) and, as it was described, a general vulnerability to stress (Barocas and Barocas 1983; Danieli 1981).

Indeed, Barocas and Barocas (1983) commented not only on the alarming number of children of survivors seeking and requiring help but also on the nature of their symptoms. They stated that offspring of Holocaust survivors "present symptomatology and psychiatric features that bear a striking resemblance to the concentration camp survivor syndrome described in the international literature" and that these children "show symptoms that would be expected if they actually lived through the Holocaust" (p. 332). That children of trauma survivors display PTSD symptoms, but to a lesser extent than parents, was also observed by Rosenheck and Nathan (1985) in their study of children of Vietnam War combat veterans. Rosenheck and Nathan termed this phenomenon "secondary traumatization."

It is interesting that after the initial reports indicating impairment in the children of Holocaust survivors came a series of studies that focused on the adaptive qualities of survivors and their children (Dimsdale 1974; Harel et al. 1988; B. Kahana et al. 1988;

Leon et al. 1981). These studies focused on the remarkable coping skills and reintegrative capacities of Holocaust survivors who demonstrated good social and family functioning, high socioeconomic achievement, good coping skills, and other personal achievements. The investigators in these studies did not find evidence of psychopathology, but they did not directly look for psychopathology or ask about it. An idea that developed from this literature was that the adaptive characteristics of the parents may have in many cases mitigated against pathology in the offspring (Helmreich 1996). And, indeed, findings of well-being in survivors were echoed by several investigators who failed to observe differences in psychopathological features of offspring compared with demographically similar subjects (Aleksandrowicz 1973; Last and Klein 1981; Rose and Garske 1987; Zlotogorski 1983).

A position taken by some describers of coping and resilience was that the findings of impairment in Holocaust survivors and their children were not generalizable to the majority of Holocaust families because the observations had been made on treatment seekers, in a relatively biased manner, and often without the use of comparison groups (see, e.g., Silverman 1987; Solkoff 1992). Although this was a valid criticism given the anecdotal nature of the clinical literature, it was becoming clear that even the more "experimental" studies of nonclinical samples of Holocaust survivors and offspring also suffered from severe methodological limitations. Solkoff (1992), in a critical review, concluded that almost no study of children of Holocaust survivors fulfilled the necessary methodological criteria related to subject selection and other experimental biases. This scathing indictment essentially rendered all conclusions in the literature—from both clinical and experimental studies of offspring—practically useless.

Although only a few groups had undertaken a comprehensive and methodologically sound approach to the study of Holocaust offspring, some intriguing findings were produced from two well-designed studies. In the first, investigators made the provocative observation that offspring of Holocaust survivors were more likely than other soldiers to develop PTSD following deployment in the Lebanon War (Solomon et al. 1988). This finding served to underscore the idea of offspring of survivors as more fragile and vulnerable. In the second study, investigators demonstrated an increased prevalence of past psychiatric disorder among an epidemiologically valid sample of Holocaust offspring compared with individuals whose parents had not survived the Holocaust (Schwartz et al. 1994). In light of these intriguing findings, we wondered about the mechanisms associated with the increased psychopathology among the offspring.

One of the ideas implicit in the descriptions of impairment of offspring was the attribution of psychiatric problems in the children of trauma survivors to the parental trauma. However, none of the findings in the literature, including Solomon et al.'s observations, directly addressed the issue of whether symptoms in offspring were the result of indirect exposure to traumatic material as described by the parents or, rather, the direct effect of parental inability to provide appropriate nurturing (which would not necessarily constitute a DSM-IV traumatic experience [American Psychiatric Association 1994]). Solomon et al. suggested that the increased incidence of PTSD after the Lebanon War in the offspring of Holocaust survivors reflected "responses that the children 'learned' from their survivor parents. For example, the second generation PTSD casualty may have more war-related nightmares than his control group peers because he had seen and heard his parents venting their emotion" (p. 867).

However, we felt that since an important risk factor for the development of PTSD is an individual's own prior history of trauma (Bremner et al. 1997; Resnick et al. 1992), a higher rate of PTSD in offspring may have reflected their own more stressful or traumatic life events in addition to the effects of parental trauma. In the absence of knowledge about each individual's stress history, we felt that it was difficult to attribute PTSD to hypothetical learned responses.

Another very important issue concerned that of heterogeneity of the parental response to trauma. There has been an implicit assumption of homogeneity in studies of Holocaust survivors and their offspring. However, our work with Holocaust survivors clearly demonstrated that although about half of survivors studied from a randomly selected sampling met the criteria for current PTSD, the other half did not. Furthermore, a significant proportion of individuals who did not have current PTSD also never met the criteria for lifetime PTSD. Similarly, although many Holocaust survivors met the diagnostic criteria for current or lifetime psychiatric disorder, many did not (Yehuda et al. 1995b). Therefore, we felt that in assessing the effects of the Holocaust on the second generation, it was not enough to simply know the trauma history of the parent; rather, we had to further explore the extent to which the Holocaust affected the parents of the children whom we studied.

Experimental Approaches in the Present Studies of Offspring of Holocaust Survivors

Our objective was to consider more carefully the mechanisms involved in the "increased vulnerability" of offspring noted in the literature. We were interested primarily in determining the generalizability of this vulnerability and also the factors that might be particularly associated with individual differences in responses of offspring. We felt it was particularly important to systematically evaluate potential differences in stressful or traumatic life events among the offspring other than those related to the parental trauma. Otherwise, we did not feel that we could necessarily attribute PTSD or other psychopathology in offspring of trauma survivors to the effect of parental trauma.

Study 1: Prevalence of Trauma Exposure, PTSD, and Other Psychiatric Disorder

In the first study (Yehuda et al. 1998b), we examined stress and trauma exposure and the prevalence of current and lifetime PTSD and other psychiatric disorders in a diverse group (consisting of both treatment seekers and community dwellers) of offspring of Holocaust survivors compared with a demographically appropriate comparison group.

Given the emphasis in the literature on the necessity of selecting a representative sample, we attempted to recruit and interview subjects from many different sources. We also performed several different comparisons in order to detect potential differences resulting from selection biases. Therefore, in addition to comparing Holocaust survivor and non–Holocaust survivor offspring, we compared Holocaust offspring not recruited from a clinical population to both the comparison subjects and the offspring recruited from a clinical population. We did not exclude treatment seekers, because excluding treatment participants from any given analysis would have biased the sample by overrepresenting non–treatment seekers. Rather, we felt that by directly comparing offspring from a clinical population with offspring recruited by other methods, we could assess the extent of bias that had been previously hypothesized as occurring.

Subjects

Offspring were defined as having been raised by at least one biological parent who survived the Nazi Holocaust. Comparison subjects were Jewish and within the same age range (i.e., 28–50 years), and they did not have a parent who was a Holocaust survivor. Subjects were recruited through a variety of methods: the clinical sample comprised offspring who had participated in short-term group psychotherapy in the Mount Sinai Specialized Treatment Program for Holocaust Survivors and Their Families and who were asked to participate in this research. The remainder of subjects were volunteers solicited from lists obtained from the Jewish community or who had responded to newspaper advertisements and community group announcements for research participants. There were no exclusions for current or past psychiatric problems (since we were interested in measuring rates of psychiatric disorders) or for any reasons other than age and non-Jewishness. The final sample consisted of 100 offspring (29 men, 71 women) and 44 comparison subjects (23 men, 21 women). The mean age ($\pm$ SD) of offspring of Holocaust survivors was 39.4 ± 6.0 and of comparison subjects, 36.9 ± 8.5. The mean years of education for offspring was 17.8 ± 1.8, and for comparison subjects, 18.9 ± 2.3. These differences were not statistically significant.

Procedure

Two scales were used to determine past and current life stress and trauma: the Trauma History Questionnaire, which is a list of 23 potentially traumatic (mostly potentially life-threatening) events, including crime, disaster, and physical and sexual assaults (B. Green, Trauma History Questionnaire, unpublished instrument and data, 1995), and the Antonovsky Life Crises Scale (Antonovsky 1979), which lists both life-threatening (e.g., having a life-threatening illness, having wartime experiences) and non–life-threatening events (e.g., family in extreme financial debt; denial of a promotion at work; feeling overwhelmed by too many responsibilities). Both scales included an open-ended question for specifying other extraordinarily stressful situations or events that "caused great suffering or tension" (Antonovsky 1979). Potentially traumatic events were then further classified as being of "low" (e.g., mugging without a weapon, motor vehicle accident without injury, sexual touching) and "high" (e.g., mugging with a weapon, motor vehicle accident with injury, rape) magnitude.

After completing both scales, subjects were asked to rank, in order of severity, events meeting part of criterion A of DSM-IV PTSD (American Psychiatric Association 1994), which were specified as "events that involved a threat to the physical integrity of self or others" (i.e., life-threatening). After ranking these events, they were asked for their most subjectively distressing event—an event that involved a response of "intense fear, helplessness, or horror" (i.e., distressing) even if that event had not been life-threatening. This question allowed us to assess PTSD symptoms in response to events that might satisfy the DSM-III-R criterion (i.e., "unusual" or "extremely distressing"), even if they would not fulfill the DSM-IV criterion of involving a threat to physical integrity.

We generated four groups based on the responses to these questions. The first group (A) indicated a life-threatening event as their most distressing one. The second group (B) indicated a non–life-threatening event as most distressing even though they had experienced a different event that could have been more appropriately considered the basis of PTSD (e.g., indicating that a divorce was more traumatic than a car accident). The third group (C) indicated a non–life-threatening event as their most distressing but had not experienced a life-threatening event. The fourth group (D) indicated that no event they had experienced was deemed subjectively distressing enough to cause fear, helplessness, and horror at the time that it occurred. (Individuals in this last group might have objectively experienced a life-threatening event but possibly minimized its impact in response to this question.)

With the first three groups, the PTSD symptoms were assessed on the basis of the most distressing event by means of the Clinician-Administered PTSD Scale (CAPS; Blake et al. 1990) and the DSM-IV PTSD symptom criteria. Other psychiatric diagnoses were made according to the DSM-IV criteria with the Structured Clinical Interview for DSM-IV (SCID; Spitzer et al. 1994).

Results and Discussion

Adult children of Holocaust survivors had a greater degree of cumulative lifetime stress compared with non-Holocaust offspring subjects (5.32 ± 0.17 vs. 2.09 ± 0.25, $t = 6.85$, $P < 0.0001$), as reflected by the Antonovsky Life Crises Scale. It is difficult to know whether offspring of Holocaust survivors actually experienced more ordinary life stress or were simply more likely to characterize these experiences as major problems or crises. However, in contrast to the higher scores on the Antonovsky Life Crises Scale for the offspring of Holocaust survivors, there were no substantial differences between the two groups in the total number of traumatic (i.e., potentially life-threatening) events as assessed by the Trauma History Questionnaire. On average, the offspring of Holocaust survivors reported 1.7 ± 1.60 such events, while the comparison subjects reported 1.98 ± 1.98 potentially life-threatening events.

Figure 5–1 illustrates the prevalence of different traumatic events among the Holocaust survivor offspring and comparison subjects. From the figure it is clear that the two groups differed slightly (nonsignificantly) in the types of events that they may have been exposed to, but essentially both groups averaged less than one high-magnitude and one low-magnitude event per subject. It

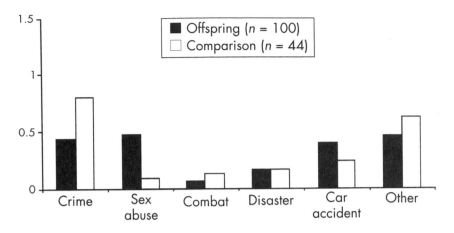

Figure 5–1.   Number of traumatic events in offspring of Holocaust survivors and comparison subjects.

can be concluded from these data that the trauma exposure for the Holocaust survivor offspring was not substantially different from that for the comparison subjects. These results were not substantially affected when treatment participants were excluded from the children of Holocaust survivors group. Furthermore, the two subgroups of offspring—the children of Holocaust survivors who were not treatment participants and those who were—did not differ in the number of traumatic events reported.

When subjects were asked to indicate their *subjectively* "most distressing" event (i.e., even if that event had not been life-threatening), Holocaust survivor offspring and comparison subjects had very different response patterns. As can be seen in Figure 5–2, the Holocaust survivor offspring were more likely than comparison subjects to endorse a non–life-threatening event (B or C) as their most distressing. This was true regardless of whether some other life-threatening event may have been present. Interestingly, there was little difference in the 34% of offspring and 40% of comparison subjects who had experienced at least one high-magnitude event that would qualify as potentially life-threatening (A and B). Again, there were no differences when treatment participants were excluded from the children of Holocaust survivors group. Further-

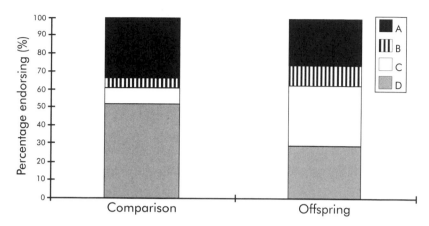

Figure 5–2. Subjectively most distressing type of event for offspring of Holocaust survivors ($n = 100$) and comparison subjects ($n = 44$). (A) A life-threatening event was most distressing. (B) A non–life-threatening event was most distressing even though there was a life-threatening event. (C) A non–life-threatening event was most distressing, with no life-threatening event. (D) No event was reported as subjectively distressing.

more, the two subgroups of offspring (those who were not treatment participants and those who were) did not differ in terms of the number of traumatic events reported.

In attempting to analyze which types of events were more frequently endorsed by both Holocaust survivor offspring and comparison subjects, it became clear that the groups tended to endorse similar life-threatening events. The exception was that a small percentage of offspring (7%) were affected by Holocaust-related stories from their parents, whereas comparison subjects did not report being subjectively distressed by experiences of family members. Although the proportion of subjects indicating these stories to be their most distressing events was small, it is important to note that when this trauma was mentioned as most distressing, it elicited lifetime PTSD for more than half of the subjects (i.e., four out of seven). Stories about the Holocaust were included as a DSM-IV event rather than a non–life-threatening event because of the inclusion of "confrontation of information of an event" in criterion A of the DSM-IV criteria.

The non–life-threatening events that Holocaust survivor off-spring endorsed as most distressing were childhood experiences relating to being a child of a Holocaust survivor, death or prolonged illness of a parent or sibling, divorce, marital difficulty, and termination of a romantic relationship. With the exception of Holocaust-related upbringing, comparison subjects typically chose similar events, but less frequently. About one-quarter of offspring who designated a non–life-threatening event as most traumatic chose an event related to their Holocaust upbringing (such as those mentioned above). About one-third (8/22) of offspring who reported non–life-threatening events related to the Holocaust as their most distressing event developed PTSD in response to the event. Thus, in both potentially life-threatening and non–life-threatening events, a substantial proportion of traumatic events in offspring was related to the Holocaust.

The other non–life-threatening events typically involved loss or separation from a significant other. In particular, offspring reported these types of losses as very upsetting. Such losses were also particularly prevalent in the responses to the Antonovsky Life Crises Scale compared with other life stressors such as loss of a job or financial difficulty.

The prevalences of current and lifetime PTSD and other psychiatric disorders are presented in Table 5–1. The prevalence of current PTSD was significantly higher ($P = 0.01$) among the children of Holocaust survivors (15%) than among the comparison subjects (2%). When treatment-seeking offspring were excluded, the difference in prevalence of current PTSD nearly remained significant ($P = 0.06$). However, the clinic and nonclinic samples were not significantly different in terms of prevalence of current PTSD. The prevalence of lifetime PTSD was significantly higher ($P = 0.004$, for lifetime) among the children of Holocaust survivors (31%) than among the comparison subjects (9%). When the clinic sample was excluded, the results were still statistically significant ($P = 0.04$). The difference between the clinic and nonclinic samples in the prevalence of lifetime PTSD was not statistically significant ($P = 0.08$) because of the reduction in sample size.

Since PTSD in offspring of Holocaust survivors included PTSD

Table 5-1. Prevalences of current and lifetime posttraumatic stress disorder (PTSD) and other psychiatric disorders among offspring of Holocaust survivors and comparison subjects

| | Comparison group (n = 44) (%) | Offspring | | | | | | | | | | | |
| | | Total sample (n = 100) | | | | Nonclinic sample (n = 64) | | | | Clinic sample (n = 36) | | | |
Diagnosis		%	χ^2	df	P	%	χ^2	df	P	%	χ^2	df	P
PTSD													
Current	2	15	5	1	0.025	12	3.6	1	...	19	0.9	1	ns
Lifetime	9	31	8	1	0.004	25	4.4	1	0	42	3	1	0.1
No disorder													
Current	91	61	14	5	0.015	66	11	4	0	53	5.9	5	ns
Lifetime	84	46	19	5	0.002	53	11	4	0	33	7.5	5	ns
Major depression													
Current	5	15				14				17			
Lifetime	7	26				22				33			
Anxiety disorder													
Current	0	10				11				8			
Lifetime	2	9				8				11			
Mood and anxiety disorder													
Current	5	9				6				14			
Lifetime	4	13				14				11			

(continued)

Table 5–1. Prevalences of current and lifetime posttraumatic stress disorder (PTSD) and other psychiatric disorders among offspring of Holocaust survivors and comparison subjects *(continued)*

| | Comparison group (n = 44) (%) | Offspring | | | | | | | | | | | |
| | | Total sample (n = 100) | | | Nonclinic sample (n = 64) | | | | Clinic sample (n = 36) | | | |
Diagnosis		%	χ^2	df	P	%	χ^2	df	P	%	χ^2	df	P
Eating disorder													
Current	0	2				0				6			
Lifetime	0	2				0				6			
Substance abuse													
Current	0	3				3				3			
Lifetime	2	4				3				6			

Note. ns = not significant.

that developed in response to Holocaust-related events, which was not the case for the comparison subjects, we compared PTSD prevalence in subjects reporting non-Holocaust events as most distressing, omitting in this analysis those who reported Holocaust-related events as most disturbing. Of the 42 offspring with a non–Holocaust-related distressing event, 45% developed lifetime PTSD. This rate was significantly higher than the 19% prevalence in the 21 comparison subjects who reported a distressing event ($\chi^2 = 4.14$, df = 1, $P < 0.05$). An additional analysis that we performed excluded all PTSD diagnoses to a non-DSM-IV trauma and only considered PTSD in the subsample of individuals endorsing a DSM-IV traumatic event (26/100 offspring and 15/44 comparison subjects). The prevalence of lifetime PTSD was more than twice as high in the offspring group—46% ($n = 12$) compared with 20% ($n = 3$) of normal subjects—who developed PTSD when only DSM-IV events were considered ($\chi^2 = 2.80$, df = 1, $P < 0.10$). Interestingly, the proportions of Holocaust survivor offspring (42%) and comparison subjects (17%) who developed "PTSD" in response to non–life-threatening events (which therefore might not be considered to meet DSM-IV criteria) were comparable to the proportions of offspring and comparison subjects who developed PTSD in response to life-threatening events.

In regard to current and lifetime psychiatric diagnoses, 38% of the offspring of Holocaust survivors, but only 5% of the comparison subjects, met the criteria for a current disorder. Similarly, 53% of the offspring, compared with 14% of the comparison subjects, met the diagnostic criteria for a lifetime psychiatric disorder. These differences were statistically significant. When treatment-seeking offspring were excluded, the prevalence of psychiatric disorder among the offspring of Holocaust survivors was reduced, but the differences between the offspring and comparison groups were still statistically significant.

Although few of the comparison subjects met the diagnostic criteria for current and lifetime PTSD and other psychiatric disorders, the actual rates of these conditions found in the present sample are consistent with base rates in larger, epidemiological studies. For example, the 9% prevalence of lifetime PTSD in the comparison population is in line with estimates of Breslau and colleagues (1991) and estimates from both the National Comorbidity Survey (Kessler et al. 1995) and the Epidemiologic Catchment Study (Davidson et al. 1991). The prevalences for depression and for anxiety in the comparison group are also compatible with published population estimates. For example, Wittchen and colleagues (1994) found a 4.9% rate of current depression and a 3.5% rate of anxiety in the general population, which are compatible with estimates of 5% current depression and 5% anxiety and mood disorder in the normal comparison subjects. It should be noted, however, that the 5% prevalence of substance use disorders in both the offspring of Holocaust survivors and the comparison subjects in our sample is considerably lower than reported national estimates of substance abuse (Anthony et al. 1994; Bucholz 1992; Judd et al. 1996).

The findings clearly demonstrate that offspring of Holocaust survivors have more current and lifetime psychiatric disorders than do comparison subjects. This is the first study to systematically evaluate the extent to which different types of recruitment influence variables related to the presence of psychopathology. However, it is clear that there was no substantial clinical distinction between these two offspring samples. When differences between Holocaust survivor offspring recruited only from the community and comparison subjects were evaluated, findings in this offspring subgroup consistently replicated the findings for the entire offspring sample, subject to a reduction in power because of the smaller sample size. Thus, the results of this study cannot be attributed to any bias introduced by inclusion of a clinical sample as has been frequently hypothesized (Solkoff 1992).

The results of this study suggested to us that children of Holocaust survivors might constitute a group "at risk" for the development of PTSD. However, the demonstration of increased rates of PTSD in this group did not in and of itself address the possible etiology (e.g., heritability, learned responses) of symptoms or the biology of the risk for PTSD. We therefore conducted some follow-up studies to address these critical issues. Our next question was, Is the increased prevalence of PTSD in offspring of Holocaust survivors directly related to parental PTSD?

Study 2: Relation of Psychiatric Symptoms in Offspring of Holocaust Survivors to Psychiatric Symptoms in the Parents

As stated earlier in this chapter, the literature has been sharply divided about whether children of Holocaust survivors are affected by the Holocaust. The results of our first study suggest that as a group, offspring are more symptomatic and have a higher prevalence of PTSD and other psychiatric disorder. However, many of the offspring of Holocaust survivors did not display evidence of significant psychopathology. The sample of offspring in our study was clearly heterogeneous.

In trying to determine some of the reasons for this marked heterogeneity, we considered the possibility that the impairment in offspring may be directly related to impairment in the parents. Although most studies of survivors and offspring assume that impairment of the trauma survivor is a direct result of the trauma exposure, it is well known that not all trauma survivors develop chronic PTSD (see, e.g., Kessler et al., Chapter 2, this volume). Indeed, although our studies have demonstrated that about half of Holocaust survivors have chronic PTSD (Yehuda et al. 1995b), most studies have tended to consider Holocaust survivors as a homogeneous group based on the experience of the Holocaust and have not subgrouped Holocaust survivors into those with and without chronic PTSD. Moreover, the children of Holocaust survivors have not been subgrouped on the basis of whether their parents had developed PTSD.

Therefore, in a second study (Yehuda et al. 1998a), we examined the relationship between PTSD characteristics of Holocaust survivors and those of their adult children in a community-based sample to determine whether differences in symptom severity or diagnostic status of parents were specifically associated with similar characteristics in their adult children.

Subjects and Recruitment

Our initial recruitment for this study began by asking the Holocaust survivors we had studied whether they would be interested in telling their children about the research project. The Holocaust survivors in these studies had all been interned in Nazi concentration camps. They were randomly selected from publicly available lists of Holocaust survivors provided by the local historical society and local synagogue membership rosters. They were invited through a mailing to participate in studies exploring the biological basis of survival and adaptation. Subjects who agreed to participate provided written informed consent and received medical clearance by one of the study physicians. None of the subjects were treatment seekers.

Almost all of the Holocaust survivors with children whom we studied were amenable to telling their children about the study. Parents were told that children interested in participating in the project may contact the local study coordinator for further information. From this effort, 22 children called us and agreed to participate in the research. Note that although the sample size is small, the subjects were recruited through a relatively nonbiased procedure.

In total, 22 Holocaust survivors (11 men, 11 women; mean age [± SD]: 67.91 ± 4.62 years; range: 58–75) and 22 adult offspring (9 men, 13 women; 37.68 ± 4.2 years; range: 31–45) were studied. The gender distribution of the parents and that of the offspring were as follows: for the 11 men, 6 of the offspring were men and 5 were women; for the 11 women, 5 of the offspring were men and 6 were women. Because the sample sizes were small, potential gender differences were not evaluated.

Eleven of the Holocaust survivors (4 men, 7 women) met the criteria for current PTSD and 11 did not; of the latter subjects, 3 met the diagnostic criteria for past PTSD. Four survivors had current major depression (2 with, 2 without PTSD), 1 (with PTSD) had dysthymia, and 3 had current generalized anxiety disorder (2 with, 1 without PTSD). Three met the criteria for past major depression. Psychiatric diagnoses were distributed evenly across gender.

Procedure

The 22 offspring were interviewed with the same structured instruments and ratings as were used in the interviews with their parents. A comprehensive trauma history was obtained with the Antonovsky Life Crises Scale and the Recent Life Events Scale (Kahana and Kahana 1982). An unstructured interview was conducted in which offspring were asked whether they felt the Holocaust had been a traumatic event in their lives. They were asked to fill out the Impact of Event Scale (Horowitz et al. 1979) and to cue their "intrusive" and "avoidance" symptoms to the Holocaust (e.g., they were asked how many times they had thought about the Holocaust in the last 7 days). They also completed the Civilian Mississippi PTSD Scale (Keane et al. 1991).

For the diagnostic portion of the interview, offspring identified traumatic events gleaned from the Antonovsky Life Crises Scale, and CAPS was used to quantify the frequency and intensity of current and lifetime PTSD. Additional information included presence of current and lifetime psychiatric diagnoses, as determined by the Structured Clinical Interview for DSM-III (Spitzer et al. 1987).

Results and Discussion

The findings show that PTSD characteristics in both Holocaust survivors and their offspring are diverse. The data also demonstrate wide-ranging associations between characteristics of trauma survivors and those of their children. There was a significant correlation between parents' and children's scores on the Civilian Mississippi PTSD Scale ($r = 0.44$; $n = 22$; $P < 0.04$). There was also a significant correlation between parents' and children's scores on the Intrusive ($r = 0.845$, $n = 13$; $P = 0.0003$), but not the Avoidance ($r = 0.11$; $n = 13$, n.s.), subscale of the Impact of Event Scale.

Offspring of Holocaust survivors were significantly more likely to develop PTSD in response to their own traumatic events if their parent had chronic PTSD. Five (1 man, 4 women) of the 22 offspring met the criteria for current or past PTSD. All 5 offspring with PTSD had parents with PTSD, but only 6 (3 men, 3 women) of the 17 offspring without PTSD had parents with PTSD. Notably, however, there was no significant difference ($t = 0.38$, $n = 21$; n.s.) in Antonovsky Life Crises Scale scores among the 5 offspring with (3.6 ± 2.7) and the 17 offspring without PTSD (3.12 ± 2.3). This suggests that having a parent with PTSD may be a risk factor for the development of PTSD in response to one's own trauma.

Interestingly, having a parent with PTSD or psychiatric diagnosis did not appear to be a risk factor for development of other psychiatric diagnoses. The relationship between parents' PTSD and children's other psychiatric diagnoses was not significant. Of the offspring with Axis I diagnoses other than PTSD (depression, panic disorder, generalized anxiety disorder, or substance abuse), four had parents with PTSD, and three had parents without PTSD. There was no significant relationship between parents' and children's diagnostic status. These findings extend the observations of Solomon and colleagues (1988) and Rosenheck and Nathan (1985), as well as the result previously reported in this chapter of increased PTSD symptoms in offspring, by clarifying that it is not the trauma exposure per se that is relevant to secondary traumatization or intergenerational responses to a traumatic event(s), but rather the posttraumatic symptoms of the parents.

The results of the first two studies, together, presented us with an interesting opportunity to obtain biological data that might be related to risk for PTSD. The results of both studies clearly suggest that children of Holocaust survivors may constitute a group at high risk for the development of PTSD and possibly other, related traumatic stress disorders. In particular, we felt it would be interesting to examine biological parameters in offspring of Holocaust survivors categorized on the basis of trauma exposure and PTSD.

Study 3: Cortisol Levels in Offspring of Holocaust Survivors

We chose to measure urinary cortisol excretion in the adult offspring of Holocaust survivors because levels of this hormone have consistently been found to be altered in trauma survivors with PTSD (Yehuda 1998; Yehuda et al. 1995a). Cortisol is a hormone that is released by the adrenal gland. In response to stress, several biological systems are activated in order to allow the body to become mobilized for the "fight or flight" reaction (Munck et al. 1984). Indeed, stress results in a coordinated sympathetic discharge that causes increases in heart rate and blood pressure, thereby allowing a greater perfusion of muscles and vital organs and increased energy to skeletal muscles by mobilizing blood glucose (Mountcastle 1973). Sympathetic nervous system activation also results in the release of catecholamines (primarily norepinephrine and epinephrine). These and other activities are part of what Cannon originally termed the "flight or fight" response (Cannon 1914). Generally, the catecholaminergic system and the hypothalamic-pituitary-adrenal axis work in tandem, and in the brain glucocorticoid and catecholamine receptors are co-localized in many areas, such as the locus coeruleus (Harfstrand et al. 1986). Thus, it is not surprising that after stress catecholamine and cortisol levels are typically highly correlated. Interestingly, however, the functions of catecholamines and cortisol are synergistic; cortisol's role in stress is to shut down sympathetic (catecholamine) activation after stress.

During stress, the brain also signals the pituitary gland to stimulate the release of cortisol from the adrenal gland. The function of cortisol in response to stress is to shut down the other biological reactions that have been turned on in order to cope with the short-term demands of a stressor (Munck et al. 1984). If cortisol did not shut off these other reactions, long-term damage to the body would ensue. Therefore, it is possible to conceptualize cortisol as an "anti-stress" hormone, because an organism's inability to produce cortisol in sufficient amounts in response to stress would have deleterious consequences.

In conditions of acute and chronic stress, and in certain types of psychiatric disorders that are associated with stress (e.g., major depression), cortisol levels are high (Mason et al. 1986; Sachar et al. 1973). In some cases, however, increased cortisol levels indicate that the HPA axis has grown resistant to the effects of cortisol (Yehuda et al. 1993). In contrast, studies in PTSD have shown that cortisol levels are lower in trauma survivors with PTSD than in healthy subjects and other psychiatric groups (Yehuda et al. 1993). However, the lower levels of cortisol appear to reflect a stress system that may actually be more responsive to external stimulation (see Yehuda 1998 for review).

A series of studies conducted in our laboratory has led us to hypothesize that low cortisol in PTSD is related to the behavioral hyperresponsiveness of trauma survivors. Since lower cortisol levels appear to be present particularly in trauma survivors with PTSD and not in trauma survivors without PTSD (see Chapter 1, this volume), we have speculated that these biological alterations reflect more than the experience of trauma exposure. Measuring cortisol levels in adult offspring of Holocaust survivors allowed us to evaluate the possibility that low cortisol levels might also be related to risk for PTSD. Support for this possibility would be obtained if adult offspring of Holocaust survivors were found to have low cortisol levels even if they had not directly experienced a traumatic event and/or developed PTSD.

Subjects and Recruitment

For the present study, we recruited subjects by placing advertisements in local newspapers around the New York metropolitan area. Many offspring also contacted us after hearing about our research through local television stories and newspaper articles or after seeing advertisements for our group therapy program. Twenty-nine offspring (4 men, 25 women) participated in the study. For this first preliminary study of cortisol levels, the primary inclusion criterion was that the subjects have at least one parent who was a Holocaust survivor. Subjects also had to be medically healthy and free of psychotropic or other medications that are known to affect cortisol levels. Comparison subjects were 11 healthy subjects (6 men, 5 women) with no current or past psychopathology.

Procedure

Clinical evaluations of trauma history and psychiatric symptoms were performed as described in the first two studies described earlier. Urine was collected beginning at 9:00 A.M. in exact 24-hour portions in 2-liter polyethylene bottles kept in freezers in the subjects' residences to ensure stability of cortisol. Collections were scheduled to occur on days when subjects planned to be home for the

24-hour period. Clinical assessments took place following the completion of the 24-hour collection, usually within the same week. Urinary free cortisol levels were determined by means of an extraction procedure and radio immunoassay kit (from Clinical Assays, Inc.).

Results and Conclusions

The following data are from work in progress, reflecting an interim analysis, and therefore should be interpreted cautiously.

Figure 5–3 shows the scatterplot of 24-hour urinary cortisol excretion in the offspring group and the control subjects. An overall ANOVA demonstrated a significant main effect of group. Mean urinary cortisol excretion (± SD) for the offspring group was

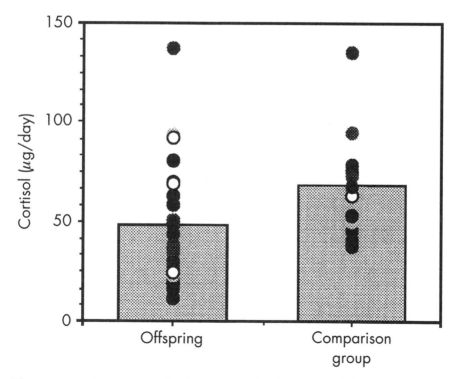

Figure 5–3. Urinary cortisol excretion in offspring of Holocaust survivors and comparison subjects.

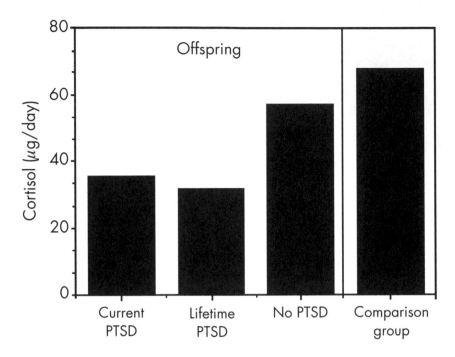

Figure 5–4. Urinary cortisol excretion in Holocaust survivor offspring with and without current and lifetime posttraumatic stress disorder (PTSD) and comparison subjects.

47.6 ± 28.6 µg/day; the mean for comparison subjects was 67.7 ± 28.4 µg/day ($t = 2.00$; df = 38; $P = 0.052$).

When offspring were further subdivided on the basis of their past and present PTSD, it became clear that PTSD status contributed to the low cortisol levels. As indicated in Figure 5–4, Holocaust offspring with lifetime PTSD ($n = 11$) had significantly lower levels of cortisol compared with offspring and comparison subjects without lifetime PTSD ($F = 5.23$; df = 2,37; $P = 0.01$). When the subset of Holocaust offspring with current PTSD ($n = 5$) were compared with Holocaust survivors without current or lifetime PTSD ($n = 18$) and comparison subjects, no main effect of group was found (possibly because of the small sample size). Rather, Holocaust offspring with current PTSD, compared with comparison subjects and Holocaust survivors without current or lifetime PTSD, showed nonsignificantly lower cortisol levels ($F = 2.14$; df = 2,31; $P = 0.13$).

When the groups were subdivided on the basis of having experienced a high-magnitude traumatic event, we found no significant differences based on trauma exposure. Offspring who had experienced a traumatic event had slightly higher cortisol levels (55.4 ± 34.1 μg/day) than did offspring who had not experienced a traumatic event of high magnitude (42.40 ± 24.3 μg/day). Cortisol levels in comparison subjects were 71.29 μg/day in those who had experienced a traumatic event vs. 63.12 μg/day in those who had not.

In sum, the results demonstrate that some offspring of Holocaust survivors have low cortisol levels. The low levels appear to be associated with lifetime PTSD in this group.

Conclusion

In considering our three studies in tandem, it can be concluded that adult children of Holocaust survivors constitute a group at high risk for PTSD and, as such, an ideal group to be studied. In particular, we can consider differences in Holocaust offspring subgrouped on the basis of their own trauma histories and psychiatric diagnoses as well as their parents' PTSD status in order to elucidate possible risk factors. Although our work is currently in preliminary stages, it may ultimately help us in identifying the biological and psychological characteristics of individuals who develop PTSD in response to traumatic events.

References

Aleksandrowicz DR: Children of concentration camp survivors, in The Child in His Family, Vol 2: The Impact of Disease and Death. Edited by Anthony EJ, Koupernik C. New York, Wiley, 1973, pp 385–392

American Psychiatric Association: Diagnostic and Statistical Manual of Mental Disorders, 4th Edition. Washington, DC, American Psychiatric Association, 1994

Anthony JC, Warner LA, Kessler RC: Comparative epidemiology of dependence on tobacco, alcohol, controlled substances, and inhalants: basic findings from the National Comorbidity Survey. Experimental and Clinical Psychopharmacology 2:244–268, 1994

Antonovsky A: Health, Stress and Coping. San Francisco, CA, Jossey-Bass, 1979

Barocas H, Barocas C: Wounds of the fathers: the next generation of Holocaust victims. International Review of Psychoanalysis 5:331–341, 1983

Blake D, Weathers F, Nagy D, et al: A clinician rating scale for current and lifetime PTSD. Behavior Therapist 13:187–188, 1990

Bremner JP, Randall P, Vermetten E, et al: MRI based measurement of hippocampal volume in posttraumatic stress disorder related to childhood physical and sexual abuse: a preliminary report. Biol Psychiatry 41:23–32, 1997

Breslau N, Davis GC, Andreski P, et al: Traumatic events and posttraumatic stress disorder in an urban population of young adults. Arch Gen Psychiatry 48:216–222, 1991

Bucholz K: Alcohol abuse and dependence from a psychiatric epidemiologic perspective. Alcohol Health Res World 16:197–208, 1992

Cannon WB: Emergency function of adrenal medulla in pain and major emotions. Am J Physiol 3:356–372, 1914

Danieli Y: Differing adaptational styles in families of survivors of the Nazi Holocaust: some implications for treatment. Child Today 10:6–10, 1981

Danieli Y: Families of survivors of the Nazi Holocaust: some short and long-term effects, in Stress and Anxiety, Vol 8. Edited by Spielberger CD, Sarason IG, Milgram NA. New York, McGraw-Hill/Hemisphere, 1982, pp 405–421

Davidson JRT, Hughes D, Blazer D, et al: Posttraumatic stress disorder in the community: an epidemiological study. Psychol Med 21:1–9, 1991

Dimsdale JG: The coping behavior of Nazi concentration camp survivors. Am J Psychiatry 131:792–797, 1974

Harel Z, Kahana B, Kahana E: Psychological well-being among Holocaust survivors and immigrants in Israel. J Trauma Stress 1:413–429, 1988

Harfstrand A, Fuxe K, Cintra A, et al: Glucocorticoid receptor immunoreactivity in monoaminergic neurons in the rat brain. Proc Natl Acad Sci U S A 83:9779–9783, 1986

Helmreich WB: Against All Odds: Holocaust Survivors and the Success-ful Lives They Made in America. New Brunswick, NJ, Transaction Publishers, 1996

Horowitz M, Wilner N, Alvarez W: Impact of Event Scale: a measure of subjective distress. Psychosom Med 41:209–218, 1979

Judd LL, Paulus MP, Wells KB, et al: Socioeconomic burden of subsyn-dromal depressive symptoms and major depression in a sample of the general population. Am J Psychiatry 153:1411–1417, 1996

Kahana B, Harel Z, Kahana E: Predictors of psychological well-being among survivors of the Holocaust, in Human Adaptation to Extreme Stress. Edited by Wilson J, Harel Z, Kahana B. New York, Plenum, 1988, pp 171–192

Kahana E, Kahana B: The Elderly Care Research Center Life Events Scale: adaptation, in Clinical and Social Psychology, Vol 1. Edited by Mangen DJ, Peterson WA. Minneapolis, University of Minnesota Press, 1982, pp 145–193

Keane TM, Caddell JM, Taylor KL: The Civilian Mississippi PTSD Scale. Boston, MA, National Center for Posttraumatic Stress Disorder, 1991

Kessler RC, Sonnega A, Bromet E, et al: Posttraumatic stress disorder in the National Comorbidity Survey. Arch Gen Psychiatry 52:1048–1060, 1995

Kestenberg JL: Psychoanalytic contributions to the problems of children of survivors from Nazi persecution. Israel Annals of Psychiatry and Related Disciplines 10:311–325, 1972

Kestenberg JS: Psychoanalyses of children of survivors from the Holo-caust: case presentation and assessment. J Am Psychoanal Assoc 28: 775–804, 1980

Kinsler F: Second generation effects of the Holocaust: the effectiveness of group therapy in the resolution of the transmission of parental trauma. Journal of Psychology and Judaism 6:53–66, 1981

Last U, Klein H: Impact de l'holocauste: transmission aux enfants de vecu des parents (Impact of the Holocaust: transmission of the parents' ex-periences to their children). L'Evolution Psychiatrique 41:375–388, 1981

Leon G, Butcher JN, Kleinman M, et al: Survivors of the Holocaust and their children. J Pers Soc Psychol 41:503–516, 1981

Mason JW, Giller EL, Kosten TR, et al: Urinary free-cortisol levels in post-traumatic stress disorder patients. J Nerv Ment Dis 174:145–159, 1986

Mountcastle ZB: Medical Physiology, 13th Edition. St Louis, MO, CV Mosby, 1973

Munck A, Guyre PM, Holbrook NJ: Physiological functions of glucocorticoids in stress and their relation to pharmacological actions. Endocr Rev 93:9779–9783, 1984

Novac A: Clinical heterogeneity in children of Holocaust survivors. Psychiatry Newsletter of the World Psychiatric Association, May 1993, pp 24–26

Rakoff VA: Long-term effect of the concentration camp experience. Viewpoints 1:17–20, 1966

Rakoff VA, Sigal JJ, Epstein N: Children and families of concentration camp survivors. Canada's Mental Health 14:24–26, 1976

Resnick HS, Kilpatrick DG, Best CL, et al: Vulnerability-stress factors in development of posttraumatic stress disorder. J Nerv Ment Dis 180: 424–430, 1992

Rose S, Garske J: Family environment, adjustment, and coping among children of Holocaust survivors: a comparative investigation. Am J Orthopsychiatry 57:332–344, 1987

Rosenheck R, Nathan P: Secondary traumatization in the children of Vietnam veterans with posttrauamtic stress disorder. Hospital and Community Psychiatry 36:538–539, 1985

Sachar EJ, Hellman L, Roffwarg HP: Disrupted 24-hour patterns of cortisol secretion in psychotic depression. Arch Gen Psychiatry 28: 19–24, 1973

Schwartz S, Dohrenwend B, Levav I: Nongenetic familial transmission of psychiatric disorders? Evidence from children of Holocaust survivors. J Health Soc Behav 35:385–402, 1994

Silverman WK: Methodological issues in the study of transgenerational effect of the Holocaust: comment on Nadler, Kav-Venaki, and Gleitman. J Consult Clin Psychol 55:125–126, 1987

Solkoff N: Children of survivors of the Nazi Holocaust: a critical review of the literature. Am J Orthopsychiatry 62:342–358, 1992

Solomon Z, Kotler M, Mikulincer M: Combat-related posttraumatic stress disorder among second-generation Holocaust survivors: preliminary findings. Am J Psychiatry 145:865–868, 1988

Spitzer RL, Williams JBW, Gibbon M: Structured Clinical Interview for DSM-III-R (SCID). New York, New York State Psychiatric Institute, Biometrics Research Unit, 1987

Trossman B: Adolescent children of concentration camp survivors. Canadian Psychiatric Association Journal 13:121–123, 1968

Waldfogel S: Physical illness in children of Holocaust survivors. Gen Hospital Psychiatry 14:267–269, 1991

Wittchen HU, Zhao S, Kesler RC: DSM-III-R generalized anxiety disorder in the National Comorbidity Survey. Arch Gen Psychiatry 51:355–364, 1994

Yehuda R: Neuroendocrinology of trauma and posttraumatic stress disorder, in Psychological Trauma. Edited by Yehuda R. Washington, DC, American Psychiatric Press, 1998, pp 97–125

Yehuda R, Resnick H, Kahana B, et al: Persistent hormonal alterations following extreme stress in humans: adaptive or maladaptive? Psychosom Med 55:287–297, 1993

Yehuda R, Kahana B, Binder-Brynes K, et al: Low urinary cortisol excretion in Holocaust survivors with posttraumatic stress disorder. Am J Psychiatry 152:982–986, 1995a

Yehuda R, Kahana B, Schmeidler J, et al: Impact of cumulative lifetime trauma and recent stress on current posttraumatic stress disorder symptoms in Holocaust survivors. Am J Psychiatry 152:1815–1818, 1995b

Yehuda R, Schmeidler J, Giller EL, et al: Relationship between posttraumatic stress disorder characteristics of Holocaust survivors and their adult offspring. Am J Psychiatry 155:841–843, 1998a

Yehuda R, Schmeidler J, Weinberger M, et al: Vulnerability to posttraumatic stress disorder in adult offspring of Holocaust survivors. Am J Psychiatry 155:1163–1171, 1998b

Zlotogorski Z: Offspring of concentration camp survivors: the relationship of perceptions of family cohesion and adaptability of levels of ego functioning. Compr Psychiatry 24:345–354, 1983

Chapter 6

Neurocognitive Risk Factors for PTSD

Scott P. Orr, Ph.D., and Roger K. Pitman, M.D.

E stimates of the prevalence of posttraumatic stress disorder (PTSD) in populations exposed to potentially traumatic events range from 1% to 15% for current PTSD and 10% to 39% for lifetime PTSD (Breslau et al. 1991; Kilpatrick and Resnick 1992; Kulka et al. 1990; Norris 1992). It is clear from these percentages that although a substantial number of individuals experiencing a traumatic event develop PTSD, most individuals do not. Explanations for why only some individuals develop PTSD include factors such as differences in the severity of the trauma, amount of social and psychological support received after the trauma, and the presence of genetic or early acquired vulnerabilities.

Individuals who develop PTSD may have experienced more severe traumatic events or a greater number of such events than were experienced by individuals who do not develop the full-blown disorder. For example, B. L. Green and colleagues (1990) reported that combat veterans exposed to grotesque death were more likely to develop PTSD than those not so exposed. Various studies have reported a positive relationship between the amount of combat exposure and presence or severity of PTSD (e.g., Kulka et al. 1990).

However, the development and severity of PTSD have also been found to differ among individuals who experienced comparably stressful events. For example, in a study of combat- related PTSD (Pitman et al. 1987), veterans with and without PTSD reported similar levels of combat exposure, yet the PTSD group showed significantly more psychiatric symptomatology and heightened

125

physiological responsivity to trauma-related experiences. This suggests that individual difference factors unrelated to the traumatic event may have contributed to the development of PTSD.

One such individual difference factor might be the amount of social and emotional support a person receives following a traumatic event (B. L. Green et al. 1990). Alternatively, differences in responses to trauma might result from genetic or acquired vulnerabilities that predispose an individual to the development of PTSD. A family history of anxiety (Davidson et al. 1985, 1989), personal history of behavioral problems (Helzer et al. 1987), neuroticism, introversion, and history of treatment for a psychological disorder (McFarlane 1988), history of early separation from caretakers, preexisting anxiety and depressive disorders, neuroticism alone, and family history of anxiety and antisocial behavior (Breslau et al. 1991) have all been found to significantly predict the development of PTSD after exposure to a stressor.

Previous Intellectual Function and Risk for PTSD

The observation that some veterans develop PTSD whereas others do not, even when exposed to comparably stressful combat experiences, led to our initial exploration for pretrauma risk factors that might predict the development of PTSD. In order to assess potential risk indicators in a manner that did not rely on retrospective and subjective reports, Pitman, Orr, and colleagues (1991) extracted information from the service military personnel and medical records of Vietnam War veterans. Information contained in these records had been collected before the veteran went to Vietnam. The records of 250 New Hampshire Vietnam combat veterans were reviewed. Of the 250 veterans whose records were reviewed, 139 individuals had a service-connected disability for a musculoskeletal wound related to combat, and 53 of these individuals had PTSD. The remaining 111 veterans had a service-connected disability for PTSD but had not been wounded. Initial screening for PTSD was accomplished with a cut-off score on the the Mississippi Scale for Combat-Related PTSD (Keane et al. 1988), followed by a diagnostic interview with the Structured Clinical Interview for DSM-III-R (SCID; Spitzer et al. 1987) in cases where PTSD was suspected.

The group of wounded veterans without PTSD was included (Pitman et al. 1991) to control for the possibility that individuals who developed PTSD simply had a higher risk of being exposed to traumatic events, rather than an increased risk for developing PTSD upon exposure. It was presumed that individuals wounded in Vietnam were likely to have had high combat exposure, such that the wounded veterans with PTSD and wounded veterans without PTSD would not have been at differential risk for exposure to traumatic events. No assumption was made regarding whether the wound was specifically responsible for the development of PTSD. From a practical standpoint, the receipt of a wound provided a means for accessing veterans' records; these records were kept locally at the regional office of the Department of Veterans Affairs in New Hampshire, and this made it more convenient to search through them to identify veterans with service-connected disabilities for musculoskeletal wounds. Nonwounded veterans with a service-connected disability for PTSD were included in this study because it seemed that they might have been especially vulnerable to the development of PTSD. If there is a reciprocal relationship between vulnerability and severity of stress, vulnerability will play a larger role in the development of PTSD to less severe stressors. It seems likely that, on average, veterans wounded in Vietnam experienced more severe combat than veterans who were not wounded. Thus, vulnerability would be expected to play a larger role in the development of PTSD in nonwounded veterans.

Several variables were extracted from the veterans' records, including the following: Armed Forces Qualifying Test (AFQT; Maier 1993) total score; AFQT Verbal and Arithmetic Reasoning subtest scores; pulse rate and blood pressure during the induction physical examination; induction physical category below "A"; and school difficulties and any positive psychiatric history item at induction.

Our primary finding was that nonwounded veterans with PTSD had lower scores on the AFQT Arithmetic Reasoning subtest and reported more difficulties in school than did veterans who never had PTSD. Scores on the AFQT Verbal subtest also tended to be lower in the nonwounded veterans with PTSD. One interpretation of these findings is that the nonwounded PTSD group had a lower preexisting intellectual ability compared with the non-PTSD group. If correct, this interpretation suggests that lower intellectual ability could be a risk factor for the development of PTSD.

Recently, Macklin and colleagues (1998) examined the relationships among performance on the AFQT, tests of current intellectual functioning, and the Clinician-Administered PTSD Scale (CAPS; Blake et al. 1995) in 90 male veterans from the Boston and Manchester Department of Veterans Affairs medical centers. They found significantly lower AFQT General Technical scores (an average of the Arithmetic Reasoning and Verbal subtests) at the time of enlistment in veterans who subsequently developed combat-related PTSD than in combat veterans who did not develop PTSD. There was a moderately strong negative Pearson correlation ($r = -0.45$, df = 88, $P < 0.001$) between AFQT General Technical score and severity of PTSD symptoms as measured by the CAPS Total score. Moreover, the AFQT General Technical score was negatively correlated ($r = -0.29$, df = 87, $P = 0.006$) with Combat Exposure Scale score (Keane et al. 1989), an indication that individuals with lower precombat intelligence scores tended to have been exposed to more severe combat. Even so, the negative relationship between AFQT General Technical score and CAPS Total score remained statistically significant when an adjustment was made for the amount of combat exposure (partial $r = -0.33$, df = 86, $P < 0.01$). This suggests that the relationship between lower premorbid intellectual ability and PTSD symptom severity is not simply a consequence of the amount of trauma exposure (i.e., that individuals with lower intellectual ability were exposed to more severe combat). McNally and Shin (1995) previously reported a negative correlation between current intellectual ability and PTSD severity. They also found that intellectual ability explained variability in PTSD severity beyond that explained by the amount of combat exposure. In fact, in that study combat exposure showed a near-zero correlation with intellectual ability.

Macklin et al. (1998) reported a respectably strong correlation ($r = 0.60$, df = 88, $P < 0.001$) between the AFQT General Technical score and current intelligence as measured by an abbreviated version of the Wechsler Adult Intelligence Scale—Revised (WAIS-R; Wechsler 1981) or Shipley Institute of Living Scale (Zachary 1991). When current intelligence was adjusted for precombat intellectual ability by means of partial correlation, current intelligence was not significantly associated (partial $r = -0.15$, df = 87, $P = 0.17$) with PTSD severity (CAPS Total score). Taken together, the findings of lower precombat intelligence scores among individuals who develop PTSD and the absence of a relationship between PTSD severity and current intelligence when adjustment is made for premorbid intellectual ability suggest that previous findings of differences between individuals with and without PTSD in current intellectual functioning (e.g., McNally and Shin 1995; Vasterling et al. 1997) reflect preexisting differences rather than a consequence of developing PTSD. This possibility obtains additional support from Vasterling and colleagues' finding that two of the WAIS-R verbal subtests (Information and Vocabulary) that differentiated Gulf War veterans with and without PTSD are often used to infer premorbid intellectual ability.

The vulnerability associated with lower intellectual ability is probably not specific to the development of PTSD. Lower intellectual ability is also related to increased risk for developing general psychological problems. Results of a large-scale study of Vietnam veterans conducted by the Centers for Disease Control (1988) indicated that veterans with lower AFQT General Technical scores at time of enlistment had a greater likelihood of reporting poorer psychological status when discharged from the military. Although lower intellectual ability may put an individual at risk for developing some psychological problems, including PTSD, after stressful experiences, it is not a risk factor for the development of any type of psychopathology.

As was pointed out by Macklin et al. (1998), hypomania (Donnelly et al. 1982) and obsessive-compulsive disorder (Rachman and Hodgson 1980, pp. 34–35) are associated with higher intellectual ability. Also, in a study of psychiatrically hospitalized children,

Hodges and Plow (1990) reported that children with a DSM-III anxiety disorder, primarily separation anxiety, had significantly lower Wechsler Intelligence Scale for Children—Revised (WISC-R; Wechsler 1974) Full Scale IQ scores than did children without an anxiety disorder, whereas there were no differences in Full Scale IQ scores between children with diagnoses of depression, oppositional disorder, or conduct disorder and those without these diagnoses.

Neurological Soft (Subtle) Signs and Risk for PTSD

The evidence for lower pretrauma intellectual ability is complemented by recent findings suggesting increased neurological compromise in individuals who develop PTSD. Gurvits and colleagues (1993) obtained a neurodevelopmental history and assessed the presence of soft (subtle) neurological signs in combat veterans with and without PTSD. These signs, which are presumably associated with subtle, nonlocalizable dysfunction of the nervous system, include frontal release reflexes, palmomental reflex, grasp reflex, and fine points of motor coordination such as walking heel to toe and performing a sequence of complex hand movements. Veterans with PTSD had substantially more soft neurological signs than did veterans without PTSD.

Strikingly, veterans with PTSD (38%) reported a larger number of developmental problems, including delayed onset of walking and speech, and learning disabilities, than did the non-PTSD group (0%). The PTSD group (39%) also reported a higher incidence of bed wetting compared with the non-PTSD group (7%). These self-reported childhood experiences suggest that at least some subtle neurological dysfunctions may have been present in the PTSD group prior to their combat experiences and could represent a risk factor for developing PTSD. Additional evidence for compromised neurological development and increased soft neurological signs in samples of combat veterans with PTSD and women with PTSD resulting from childhood sexual abuse has recently been reported by Gurvits and colleagues (1997).

Hippocampal Volume Reduction and PTSD

The presence of neurological soft signs implies the existence of underlying neurological compromise and raises the possibility that there are structural differences in the brains of individuals with and without PTSD. In fact, recent studies using magnetic resonance imaging (MRI) have found that hippocampal volumes in individuals with PTSD were smaller than those in individuals without PTSD. Bremner and colleagues (1995) reported right hippocampal volume to be 8% smaller in Vietnam veterans with combat-related PTSD who were compared with a non–trauma-exposed group matched on several demographic and physical characteristics and on number of years of alcohol abuse. In a study that combined MRI and magnetic resonance spectroscopy, Schuff and colleagues (1997) noted that right hippocampal volumes in veterans with combat-related PTSD were 6% smaller than those in a non–trauma-exposed comparison group. Although the group difference was not significant, because the sample sizes were small, the effect size was substantial (0.71). Spectroscopic imaging revealed less of the amino acid N-acetyl aspartate (NAA) in the right hippocampi of the PTSD group, a finding that suggests lower neuronal density in this structure in these individuals.

Two studies of adults who experienced childhood abuse have also reported smaller hippocampal volumes in trauma-exposed individuals. Bremner and colleagues (1997) reported left hippocampal volumes to be 12% smaller in a mixed sample of 17 women and men with PTSD resulting from childhood physical and/or sexual abuse who were compared with 17 nonabused individuals. Stein and colleagues (1997) found left hippocampal volumes to be 5% smaller in 21 women with severe childhood sexual abuse who were compared with 21 women who had not been abused. Stein et al. noted that 15 of the 21 abused women met the DSM-IV criteria for current PTSD, and most also met the criteria for a dissociative disorder. These studies are suggestive of a relationship between PTSD and smaller hippocampal volume. However, because the subjects in the comparison groups had not been exposed to trauma, it is possible that trauma exposure, rather than PTSD, accounted for the findings.

Results from a study of combat-related PTSD reported by Gurvits and colleagues (1996) indicated that hippocampal volumes in trauma-exposed individuals who did not have PTSD were not reduced. Gurvits et al. found significantly smaller left (26%) and right (22%) hippocampal volumes in a sample of seven combat veterans with PTSD, compared with seven combat veterans without PTSD. Total hippocampal volume, PTSD severity as measured by CAPS Total score, and amount of combat exposure were highly intercorrelated (correlations were calculated across both groups). Because the PTSD and comparison groups had both been exposed to combat, the observed differences in hippocampal volumes could not be attributed to the mere fact of combat exposure. However, severity of the trauma, as indexed by the Combat Exposure Scale, differed between the groups and showed a strong negative linear relationship with total hippocampal volume ($r = -.72$, df $= 12$, $P < 0.01$). Consequently, differences in either severity of combat-related trauma or the presence of PTSD could explain the smaller hippocampal volumes in the PTSD group.

The evidence presented in this section thus far supports a relationship between smaller hippocampal volume and severity of trauma exposure and/or PTSD symptomatology. However, the causal links that form the basis of this association are unclear. One possibility is that smaller volumes in the PTSD group represent hippocampal atrophy resulting from high levels of stress hormones caused by exposure to a traumatic event. Research with animals has clearly demonstrated that exposure to severe stressors can produce a measurable reduction in hippocampal volume (see, e.g., Sapolsky et al. 1985; Uno et al. 1989; Watanabe et al. 1992). In considering this explanation, it should be noted that, to date, emerging evidence does not support the idea that stress hormones are elevated in the immediate aftermath of trauma in those most likely to develop PTSD (see Chapter 8, this volume). Hippocampal atrophy and PTSD may both be consequences of exposure to severe stress and thus may have no direct link to each other. It is also possible that severe stress causes PTSD and that the adverse biological, psychological, and social consequences of PTSD are responsible for hippocampal atrophy. Alternatively, smaller hippocampal volume could represent a risk factor for PTSD. Smaller hippocampi might result from genetic determinants or impaired neurological development. As was discussed earlier, there is clear support for the latter possibility (Gurvits et al. 1993, 1997). Furthermore, Gurvits et al. (1996) found that in addition to having smaller hippocampal volumes, five of the seven veterans with PTSD, but none of the non-PTSD veterans, reported a history of enuresis, a possible indicator of delayed neurodevelopment.

The hippocampus has a role in declarative, but not nondeclarative, memory (for review, see Squire 1992). Some studies (Bremner et al. 1995; Gurvits et al. 1996) have reported a significant negative relationship between hippocampal volume and performance on memory tasks. These findings raise the possibility that impairments in content-independent (McNally 1996) declarative memory, often observed in PTSD (e.g., McNally et al. 1995; Sutker et al. 1991; Yehuda et al. 1995), result from smaller hippocampi. Moreover, memory that does not depend on hippocampal integrity—that is, implicit or nondeclarative memory—does not appear to be impaired in individuals with PTSD (Amir et al. 1997; McNally and Amir 1996).

One might speculate that if poorer memory results from smaller hippocampi, and the smaller hippocampi existed prior to developing PTSD or being exposed to trauma, memory difficulties should also have been premorbidly present. As noted earlier, there is clear evidence for lower premorbid intellectual ability in individuals who develop PTSD. Given that memory plays an important role in intellectual development, the quality of this cognitive function will directly influence performance on many tasks used to assess intellectual ability. Thus, memory impairment resulting from compromised hippocampal development might explain the reduced premorbid intellectual ability in PTSD. Alternatively, impaired memory and smaller hippocampal volumes could result from severe stress, the development of PTSD, or both. A prospective study in which hippocampal volume is assessed prior to trauma exposure (or very soon afterward) and before the development of PTSD could illuminate whether reduced hippocampal size represents a risk factor for, or a consequence of, PTSD.

There is also evidence for hippocampal involvement in conditioning and extinction. In their discussion of this topic, Falls and Davis (1995) noted that rats with hippocampal lesions showed stronger conditioned fear, as evidenced by more rapid acquisition of an avoidance response to an auditory cue paired with shock, as well as more fear behavior following acquisition, than did non-lesioned rats (Antelman and Brown 1972). As a risk factor for PTSD, smaller hippocampal volume (or lower neuronal density) might predispose an individual to the acquisition of stronger and/or more persistent emotional responses when exposed to a traumatic event. Conditioning theory has been used as an explanatory framework for the findings of heightened physiological reactivity to reminders of the traumatic event in individuals with PTSD (Keane et al. 1985; Kolb and Multalipassi 1982; Pitman 1988). However, it is unclear whether this heightened reactivity to trauma reminders is a consequence of stronger conditioning, which would produce a more persistent emotional response, or a consequence of the failure to extinguish an acquired emotional response. Similarly, whether hippocampal lesions facilitate aversive conditioning or interfere with extinction remains unresolved (Falls and Davis 1995). If smaller hippocampal volume is a risk factor for PTSD, it would be most interesting to examine its relationship with condition-ability in this disorder.

Causal Inferences

The evidence for poorer pretrauma intellectual ability (Macklin et al. 1998; Pitman et al. 1991) and compromised neurodevelopmental history (Gurvits et al. 1993, 1997) supports the existence of one or more neurocognitive risk factors for developing PTSD. This vulnerability might compromise an individual's ability to adapt psychologically and emotionally to a traumatic event at the time of its occurrence or during the ensuing weeks, months, or years. The extent to which impairment in neurocognitive function plays a direct or indirect role in the development of PTSD or is merely an epi-phenomenon is unclear. It could represent an innate, biologically based deficiency that is relatively independent from environmen-tal influences, or it might be a consequence of pathogenic expe-riences such as physical or emotional abuse. Indeed, some individuals who develop PTSD are more likely to report an early history of physical and/or sexual abuse than are individuals who do not develop PTSD (Bremner et al. 1993; Donovan et al. 1996). Physical and sexual abuse have been found to be associated with impaired neurological and cognitive functioning in children (Davies 1979; Einbender and Friedrich 1989; A. H. Green et al. 1981; Ito et al. 1993; Teicher et al. 1997), but the causal direction of this as-sociation is not clear. Rather than being a consequence of abuse, impaired neurological and cognitive functioning could increase the likelihood that a child will be a victim of abuse (see, e.g., Huessy 1989; Sandgrund et al. 1974).

Impaired neurocognitive ability might indirectly influence the risk for developing PTSD by increasing the likelihood that an indi-vidual will be exposed to severe stressors. B. L. Green and col-leagues (1990) found that a lower educational level at the time of enlistment predicted the subsequent development of PTSD. Be-cause individuals who were younger and less well educated were exposed to more severe combat, it is possible that the higher trauma severity was responsible for the development of PTSD. Lower neurocognitive ability could be responsible for poorer edu-cational achievement; individuals who struggle with schoolwork are more likely to drop out or to decide not to pursue higher educa-tion. Thus, the assignment to high-risk military occupations that require little educational experience could be an indirect result of poorer neurocognitive abilities.

Sutker and colleagues (1994) reported a high prevalence of life-time and current PTSD in veterans deployed to the Persian Gulf during Operation Desert Storm who worked in graves registration. The mean current estimated WAIS-R score for graves registration veterans deployed to the war zone was 91.8 (SD = 9.7); the mean score was 90.2 (SD = 10.4) for those not deployed and in whom the incidence of PTSD was 0%. In a separate study of Operation Desert

Storm veterans, Vasterling and colleagues (1997) reported a mean WAIS-R score of 97.9 (SD = 10.7) for a group of veterans free from psychopathology. The comparably low intelligence scores in the deployed and nondeployed veterans performing graves registration suggest that the low scores for veterans who had been deployed to the war zone, among whom there was a high incidence of PTSD, were indicative of preexisting abilities and not a consequence of being exposed to war-zone trauma or the development of PTSD. Assignment to graves registration duty was voluntary. However, one cannot help but wonder about possible selection bias(es) that may have resulted in veterans with somewhat lower intellectual ability either choosing or being selected from among volunteers to perform graves registration duty. Once assigned, these individuals were at increased risk for exposure to severe trauma and the subsequent development of PTSD.

Conclusion

The research discussed above suggests that lower neurocognitive ability may have a twofold impact on the development of PTSD. First, lower cognitive ability appears to be associated with an increased vulnerability for developing PTSD upon exposure to a traumatic event (e.g., Macklin et al. 1998; Pitman et al. 1991). The way this vulnerability might influence the development of PTSD is unclear. It could determine how an individual encodes the traumatic event or copes with the emotional and psychological aftermath (Basoglu et al. 1994; Hamilton 1982; Schnurr et al. 1993). Second, lower cognitive ability may put some individuals at increased risk of being exposed to highly stressful events (e.g., B. L. Green et al. 1990; Sutker et al. 1994). Thus, the most vulnerable individuals may also have the greatest risk of being exposed to traumatic events.

This, of course, does not mean that people with high cognitive function cannot develop PTSD. Indeed, it is also possible that lower neurocognitive ability has no direct or indirect influence on the risk of developing PTSD. It may simply accompany some third, as yet unknown, factor that actually determines the degree of risk. This latter possibility clearly has implications for the theoretical understanding of PTSD and the factors that may put an individual at risk for developing the disorder. Aside from the theoretical questions, the fact that individuals who develop PTSD are likely to have lower premorbid neurocognitive ability has important implications for the study of current neurocognitive functions in this disorder.

References

Amir N, McNally RJ, Wiegartz PS: Implicit memory bias for threat in posttraumatic stress disorder. Cognitive Therapy Research 20:625–635, 1997

Antelman SM, Brown TS: Hippocampal lesions and shuttlebox avoidance behavior: a fear hypothesis. Physiol Behav 9:15–20, 1972

Basoglu M, Paker M, Paker O, et al: Psychological effects of torture: a comparison of tortured with nontortured political activists in Turkey. Am J Psychiatry 151:76–81, 1994

Blake DD, Weathers FW, Nagy LM, et al: The development of a clinician-administered PTSD scale. J Trauma Stress 8:75–90, 1995

Bremner JD, Southwick SM, Johnson DR, et al: Childhood physical abuse and combat-related posttraumatic stress disorder in Vietnam veterans. Am J Psychiatry 150:235–239, 1993

Bremner JD, Randall P, Scott TM, et al: MRI-based measurement of hippocampal volume in patients with combat-related posttraumatic stress disorder. Am J Psychiatry 152:973–981, 1995

Bremner JD, Randall P, Vermetten E, et al: Magnetic resonance imaging–based measurement of hippocampal volume in posttraumatic stress disorder related to childhood physical and sexual abuse—a preliminary report. Biol Psychiatry 41:23–32, 1997

Breslau N, Davis G, Andreski P, et al: Traumatic events and posttraumatic stress disorder in an urban population of young adults. Arch Gen Psychiatry 48:216–222, 1991

Centers for Disease Control: Vietnam Experiences Study. Health status of Vietnam veterans I: psychosocial characteristics. JAMA 259:2701–2707, 1988

Davidson JRT, Swartz M, Storck M, et al: A diagnostic and family study of posttraumatic stress disorder. Am J Psychiatry 142:90–93, 1985

Davidson JRT, Smith R, Kudler H: Familial psychiatric illness in chronic posttraumatic stress disorder. Compr Psychiatry 30:339–345, 1989

Davies RK: Incest: some neuropsychiatric findings. Int J Psychiatry Med 9:117–121, 1979

Donnelly EF, Murphy DL, Goodwin FK, et al: Intellectual functioning in primary affective disorder. Br J Psychiatry 140:633–636, 1982

Donovan BS, Padin-Rivera E, Dowd T, et al: Childhood factors and war zone stress in chronic PTSD. J Trauma Stress 9:361–368, 1996

Einbender AJ, Friedrich WN: Psychological functioning and behavior of sexually abused girls. J Abnorm Psychol 57:155–157, 1989

Falls WA, Davis M: Behavioral and physiological analysis of fear inhibition: extinction and conditioned inhibition, in Neurobiological and Clinical Consequences of Stress: From Normal Adaptation to PTSD. Edited by Friedman MJ, Charney DS, Deutch AY. Philadelphia, PA, JB Lippincott–Raven, 1995, pp 177–202

Green AH, Voeller K, Gaines R, et al: Neurological impairment in maltreated children. Child Abuse Negl 5:129–134, 1981

Green BL, Grace MC, Lindy JD, et al: Risk factors for PTSD and other diagnoses in a general sample of Vietnam veterans. Am J Psychiatry 147:729–733, 1990

Gurvits TV, Lasko NB, Schachter SC, et al: Neurological status of Vietnam veterans with chronic posttraumatic stress disorder. J Neuropsychiatry Clin Neurosci 5:183–188, 1993

Gurvits TV, Shenton ME, Hokama H, et al: Magnetic resonance imaging study of hippocampal volume in chronic, combat-related posttraumatic stress disorder. Biol Psychiatry 40:1091–1099, 1996

Gurvits TV, Gilbertson MW, Lasko NB, et al: Neurological status of combat veterans and adult survivors of sexual abuse PTSD. Ann N Y Acad Sci 821:468–471, 1997

Hamilton V: Cognition and stress: an information processing model, in Handbook of Stress: Theoretical and Clinical Aspects. Edited by Golberger L, Breznitz S. New York, Free Press, 1982, pp 105–120

Helzer JE, Robins LN, McEvoy L: Post-traumatic stress disorder in the general population: findings of the Epidemiologic Catchment Area survey. N Engl J Med 317:1630–1634, 1987

Hodges K, Plow J: Intellectual ability and achievement in psychiatrically hospitalized children with conduct, anxiety, and affective disorders. J Consult Clin Psychol 58:589–595, 1990

Huessy HR: PTSD and sexually abused children (letter). J Am Acad Child Adolesc Psychiatry 29:298–299, 1989

Ito Y, Teicher MH, Glod CA, et al: Increased prevalence of electrophysiological abnormalities in children with psychological, physical, and sexual abuse. J Neuropsychiatry Clin Neurosci 5:401–408, 1993

Keane TM, Fairbank JA, Caddell JM, et al: A behavioral approach to assessing and treating post-traumatic stress disorder, in Trauma and Its Wake: The Study and Treatment of Post-Traumatic Stress Disorder. Edited by Figley CR. New York, Brunner/Mazel, 1985, pp 257–294

Keane TM, Caddell JM, Taylor KL: Mississippi Scale for Combat-Related Posttraumatic Stress Disorder: three studies in reliability and validity. J Consult Clin Psychol 56:85–90, 1988

Keane TM, Fairbank JA, Caddell JM, et al: Clinical evaluation of a measure to assess combat exposure. Psychological Assessment: A Journal of Consulting and Clinical Psychology 1:53–55, 1989

Kilpatrick D, Resnick H: PTSD associated with exposure to criminal victimization in clinical and community populations, in Posttraumatic Stress Disorder: DSM-IV and Beyond. Edited by Davidson JRT, Foa EB. Washington, DC, American Psychiatric Press, 1992, pp 113–143

Kolb LC, Multalipassi LR: The conditioned emotional response: a subclass of the chronic and delayed post-traumatic stress disorder. Psychiatric Annals 12:979–987, 1982

Kulka RA, Schlenger WE, Fairbank JA, et al: Trauma and the Vietnam War Generation: Report of Findings From the National Vietnam Veterans Readjustment Study. New York, Brunner/Mazel, 1990

Macklin ML, Metzger LJ, Litz BT, et al: Lower pre-combat intelligence is a risk factor for post-traumatic stress disorder. J Consult Clin Psychol 66:323–326, 1998

Maier MH: Military Aptitude Testing: The Past Fifty Years (DMDC Technical Report 93–007). Monterey, CA, Personnel Testing Division, Defense Manpower Data Center, 1993

McFarlane AC: The longitudinal course of posttraumatic morbidity: the range of outcomes and their predictors. J Nerv Ment Dis 176:30–40, 1988

McNally RJ: Cognitive bias in the anxiety disorders. Nebr Symp Motiv 43:211–250, 1996

McNally RJ, Amir N: Perceptual implicit memory for trauma-related information in posttraumatic stress disorder. Cognition and Emotion 10:555–556, 1996

McNally RJ, Shin LM: Association of intelligence with severity of posttraumatic stress disorder symptoms in Vietnam combat veterans. Am J Psychiatry 152:936–938, 1995

McNally RJ, Lasko NB, Macklin ML, et al: Autobiographical memory disturbance in combat-related posttraumatic stress disorder. Behav Res Ther 33:619–630, 1995

Norris FH: Epidemiology of trauma: frequency and impact of different potentially traumatic events on different demographic groups. J Consult Clin Psychol 60:409–418, 1992

Pitman RK: Post-traumatic stress disorder, conditioning, and network theory. Psychiatric Annals 18:182–189, 1988

Pitman RK, Orr SP, Forgue DF, et al: Psychophysiologic assessment of posttraumatic stress disorder imagery in Vietnam combat veterans. Arch Gen Psychiatry 44:970–975, 1987

Pitman RK, Orr SP, Lowenhagen MJ, et al: Pre-Vietnam contents of posttraumatic stress disorder veterans' service medical and personnel records. Compr Psychiatry 32:416–422, 1991

Rachman SJ, Hodgson RJ: Obsessions and Compulsions. Englewood Cliffs, NJ, Prentice-Hall, 1980

Sandgrund A, Gaines RW, Green AH: Child abuse and mental retardation: a problem of cause and effect. American Journal of Mental Deficiency 79:327–330, 1974

Sapolsky RM, Krey LC, McEwen BS: Prolonged glucocorticoid exposure reduces hippocampal neuron number: implications for aging. J Neurosci 5:1222–1227, 1985

Schnurr PP, Rosenberg SD, Friedman MJ: Change in MMPI scores from college to adulthood as a function of military service. J Abnorm Psychol 102:288–296, 1993

Schuff N, Marmar CR, Weiss DS, et al: Reduced hippocampal volume and N-acetyl aspartate in posttraumatic stress disorder. Ann N Y Acad Sci 821:516–520, 1997

Spitzer RL, Williams JBW, Gibbon M, et al: Structured Clinical Interview for DSM-III-R. New York, New York State Psychiatric Institute, Biometrics Research Unit, 1987

Squire LR: Memory and the hippocampus: a synthesis from findings with rats, monkeys, and humans. Psychol Rev 99:195–231, 1992

Stein MB, Koverla C, Hannah C, et al: Hippocampal volume in women victimized by childhood sexual abuse. Psychol Med 27:951–959, 1997

Sutker PB, Winstead DK, Galina ZH, et al: Cognitive deficits and psychopathology among former prisoners of war and combat veterans of the Korean conflict. Am J Psychiatry 148:67–72, 1991

Sutker PB, Uddo M, Brailey K, et al: Psychopathology in war-zone deployed and nondeployed Operation Desert Storm troops assigned to graves registration duties. J Abnorm Psychol 103:383–390, 1994

Teicher MH, Ito Y, Glod CA, et al: Preliminary evidence for abnormal cortical development in physically and sexually abused children. Ann N Y Acad Sci 821:160–175, 1997

Uno H, Tarara R, Else J, et al: Hippocampal damage associated with prolonged and fatal stress in primates. J Neurosci 9:1705–1711, 1989

Vasterling JJ, Brailey K, Constans JI, et al: Assessment of intellectual resources in Gulf War veterans: relationship to PTSD. Assessment 4:51–59, 1997

Watanabe Y, Gould E, McEwen BS: Stress induces atrophy of apical dendrites of hippocampal CA3 pyramidal neurons. Brain Res 588:341–345, 1992

Wechsler D: Manual for the Wechsler Intelligence Scale for Children—Revised. New York, Psychological Corporation, 1974

Wechsler D: WAIS-R Manual: Wechsler Adult Intelligence Scale—Revised. New York, Harcourt Brace, 1981

Yehuda R, Keefe RSE, Harvey PD, et al: Learning and memory in combat veterans with posttraumatic stress disorder. Am J Psychiatry 152:137–139, 1995

Zachary RA: Shipley Institute of Living Scale: Revised Manual. Los Angeles, CA, Western Psychological Services, 1991

Chapter 7

Psychophysiological Expression of Risk Factors for PTSD

Arieh Y. Shalev, M.D.

Risk Factors and Psychophysiological Research

A risk factor is "an attribute, or habit, or exposure to some environmental hazard that leads the individual concerned to have a greater likelihood of developing an illness" (Oxford Medical Dictionary 1996). Many risk factors for PTSD have been described in this volume as well as in other sources. They include biological (e.g., genetic [True et al. 1993]), psychological (e.g., neuroticism [McFarlane 1989]), and biographical (e.g., parental violence [North and Smith 1992]) factors. Some risk factors increase the likelihood of exposure to traumatic events, others predispose to developing PTSD upon exposure, and still others are linked with the onset of chronic PTSD (Breslau and Davis 1992).

The clinical relevance of a risk factor strongly depends on its expression, measurement, and specificity. Some risk factors currently escape all measurement (e.g., a genetic constellation), others are not expressed before the traumatic event, and still others are expressed but do not have enough power to effectively detect PTSD. Hence, the very ambitious goal of forecasting and eventually preventing PTSD by identifying subjects at risk (e.g., preventing neurotic soldiers from being exposed to heavy combat) is often limited by inadequate specificity and sensitivity of the predictors (in this case, neuroticism's being widespread and predicting a small amount of the total causation of combat-related PTSD). A better understanding of the disorder, however, can reasonably be gained from studying its risk factors.

Based on the above definition and caveats, psychophysiological risk factors for PTSD can be defined as the *patterns* of body responses that predispose to developing the disorder. It should be stated, however, that the peripheral measures that are used in psychophysiological research (e.g., heart rate) are mere expressions of an underlying physiological activity that, in its turn, reflects various levels of neurohormonal regulation resulting from the combined effect of biological, psychological, and biographical (e.g., learning) factors. Psychophysiological changes, therefore, must not be confused with the underlying patterns of physiological activity that they express. For example, an increase in heart rate may result from not only increased sympathetic activation or decreased parasympathetic control but also the more remote constructs of sensitization, learning, or conditioning. Accuracy in inferring such constructs from "crude" psychophysiological measures is crucial.

In this chapter, therefore, I begin by defining basic psychophysiological dimensions. I then describe some underlying patterns and critically discuss the validity of these patterns and their relevance to PTSD.

Psychophysiological Measures

Psychophysiology has been defined as "the study of the interactions and the relationship between psychological and physiological processes" (Orr 1990, p. 137). In practice, the term *psychophysiology* refers to the study of peripheral measures such as heart rate, blood pressure, skin conductance, and muscular activity. These measures have the advantage of being both reliable and noninvasive. Their major disadvantage is that they are distal to neuronal and hormonal regulation.

Baseline Activity

At a first level, psychophysiological studies evaluate "baseline" or "resting" activity. These indices can also be measured before and after challenge or activation tests. Such an approach is subject to criticism in that the presumably neutral resting periods, during which "baseline" measures are recorded, are often contaminated by expectations (e.g., expecting startling tones) and appraisal (e.g., a sound-proof laboratory may be threatening to some). Moreover, body posture, external heat, noise, and monotony are frequent confounds of baseline measurement. However, baseline assessments are necessary in that without them no other measurement can be adequately interpreted.

Response to Challenge

Challenge tests provide a measure of reactivity. Types of challenge involved in such tests are physiological challenge (e.g., riding a bike), psychological challenge (e.g., exposure to cues that remind one of the trauma), physical challenge (e.g., loud tones), and chemical challenge (e.g., infusion of lactate). An advantage of challenge techniques is that, beyond comparisons between groups, each subject is used as his or her own control (e.g., before and during a test) and a "within-subject" repeated-measures design applies. Optimally, a group–by–repeated measures interaction is sought such that belonging to a particular group affects the way in which individuals respond to the task.

More Complex (and Hypothetical) Constructs

Baseline activity, resting levels, and response to challenge are subject to generalizations at higher levels of complexity. These generalizations not only involve theory and interpretation but also provide a context for describing stable patterns of behavior, which are better candidates for becoming risk factors. The following constructs are of particular relevance for PTSD: reactivity; conditionability; rehearsal, habituation, and extinction; anxiety; and stimulus discrimination.

Reactivity

Reactivity describes the link between the intensity of a challenge and the magnitude of the response. Reactivity is a generalization from the study of responses to challenge, in which the basic assumption is that a value or a function can be assigned to the link between challenge and response and that this function varies between individuals. Increased reactivity to challenge has been found in patients with chronic PTSD. Yet, for this construct to become a risk factor for PTSD, it must precede the disorder. Consequently, direct evidence for the existence of risk factors can be derived only from measurement performed before the onset of the disorder. Indirectly, and less convincingly, there should at least be a pattern of increased responses to a variety of stimuli, including ones that are not related to content or the antecedents of the current PTSD. Alternatively, reactivity can be a feature of PTSD, which develops along with the disorder.

Conditionability

Conditionability is the extent to which an individual or a group of individuals are prone to acquire conditioned responses upon exposure to conditioning events. Heightened conditionability may increase the risk for developing PTSD after traumatic exposure. Yet, for conditionability to become a risk factor for PTSD, it must also preexist the trauma, or at least manifest itself in a variety of exposure conditions. Hence, the psychophysiological demonstration of heightened conditionability in PTSD requires that the acquisition of conditioned response to nontraumatic stimuli be evaluated.

Rehearsal, Habituation, and Extinction

Although conditionability may explain the acquisition of strong conditioned responses, the hallmark of PTSD is, in fact, the persistence of such responses over time (Kolb 1987). Obviously, stronger conditioning is less likely to be forgotten, but this alone may not explain why the response persists. Putative explanations for persistence include *rehearsal* (i.e., through repeated recollection of the traumatic event [Baum 1990]), *secondary reinforcement* (e.g., through rewarded avoidance of reminders of the trauma [Keane et al. 1985]), and *ineffective extinction* (which is possibly a neurobiological attribute [Charney et al. 1993]). Physiological evidence for rehearsal must be based, in part, on early responses to recollections of the traumatic event (see discussion of cues to trauma later in this chapter). Habituation and extinction are difficult to measure in the context of complex psychological phenomena; yet, extinction can be measured directly, in experimental conditions, and may also be inferred from studies of startle habituation in PTSD (see discussion later in this chapter).

Anxiety

Anxiety, for the purposes of this discussion, is considered to be distinct from fear, with support for such a differentiation derived from studies of responses to startle in PTSD (e.g., Davis et al. 1997; Morgan et al. 1995, 1996). Anxiety, in this context, is expressed by an increase in auditory startle response in the presence of unsettling contextual cues (e.g., walking in a dark alley), whereas fear is represented by an increased startle in the presence of a threatening object (e.g., a gun). The neuronal mediations of such "anxiety" and "fear" have been described, and their relevance to PTSD lies in the fact that if PTSD is mediated as "anxiety," then its treatment by specific, desensitizing fear-conditioned responses (e.g., to the gun) may not address the appropriate dimension of the disorder.

Stimulus Discrimination and Evaluation

PTSD patients frequently extend their negative emotional reactions to cues that were not present during the traumatic event but are present during their daily lives (e.g., noisy environment, bad news). How accurately PTSD patients can discriminate threatening from nonthreatening information, and whether such fuzziness in perception and discrimination contributes to the occurrence of PTSD, may be inferred from psychophysiological studies, as discussed in the next section.

Critical (or Sensitive) Period

The concept of sensitive, or "critical," periods has been neglected in studies of PTSD, hence its extended discussion here. While clearly recognizing the effect of external environment on the central nervous system (CNS), most PTSD studies have used either a simplified "stress" model, in which the causation of PTSD is explained in large part by the "traumatic event," or a slightly more sophisticated "stress-vulnerability" model, which admits "prior variables." In addition, the disease model has been used extensively, such that the maladaptive development that follows traumatic events has been associated with destruction and neuropathology (e.g., loss of hippocampal neurons). Clearly, the consequences of exposure can also represent a novelty, a process of learning and differentiation, to which a social context (e.g., desirability of remaining competitive and "happy") assigns a negative value.

Differentiation is always associated with a degree of loss and with narrowing of potential. Imprinting of parental choice in birds, which is usually regarded as the archetypal form of behavioral differentiation, consists of restriction of choices, such that unrelated adults are less likely to be taken for parents. Commenting on such occurrence, Bateson (1984) suggested that "imprinting is a pre-emptive self terminating process in the sense that it narrows social preferences to that which is familiar, and therefore *tends to prevent fresh experience from further modifying those social preferences*" (p. 59; emphasis added).

In PTSD and trauma, clearly, social preferences and social appraisal are modified by experience in a decisive way. Threat is preferentially perceived (Zeitlin and McNally 1991) and previously joyful activities are avoided. The traumatized individual becomes attached to his or her traumatic past. Such learning becomes the source of lifetime misery for some. Yet, learning it may be. Within this learning model, a central question concerns whether there exists a critical (or sensitive) period, during which such narrowing down, or "pruning," of neurobehavioral options operates. Theoretical questions are whether one should assume a transient increase in neuronal plasticity during such a "critical period," and what might mediate such "openness to change." Psychophysiological dimensions of PTSD can be used as indicators of a critical period if they do not exist shortly after the traumatic event and later become pronounced as the subject develops PTSD.

Psychophysiological Findings in PTSD

Baseline Activity

Symptoms of sympathetic activation "resembling the effects of an injection of adrenaline" have been described among impaired combat veterans of World Wars I and II. However, findings of basal sympathetic activity in PTSD are diverse (e.g., Southwick et al. 1993). Elevated resting heart rate has been reported in PTSD by some authors, typically while patients were expecting a stressful task (see discussion later in this section). Other studies have failed to find differences in baseline heart rate and basal sympathetic activity between PTSD and control subjects. Importantly, when PTSD subjects were maintained in a supine position for 30 minutes, their heart rate, blood pressure, and plasma norepinephrine level did not differ from those of control subjects (McFall et al. 1992). Hence, it is generally believed (e.g., Prins et al. 1995) that baseline heart rate and baseline sympathetic activity may not be higher in individuals with PTSD.

Activity During Special Circumstances

Nontraumatic Stress

Exposure to a nontraumatic, yet stressful situation seems to increase heart rate and sympathetic activation in individuals with PTSD. Elevated heart rate and blood pressure were found in Vietnam War veterans with PTSD who were waiting for medical treatment in an emergency room and in veterans triaged in a non-research environment for medical treatment (Gerardi et al. 1994). Resting heart rate was also found to be higher in Vietnam veterans who were expecting psychophysiological testing of their responses to a trauma. Summarizing 10 psychophysiological studies of PTSD, McFall and Murburg (1994) described higher resting heart rate in patients with PTSD ($n = 151$) compared with a mixed sample of combat-exposed and non–combat-exposed control subjects ($n = 134$) (77.3 beats per minute [bpm] vs. 68.3 bpm). The mean heart rate for the group of PTSD patients, however, did not differ significantly from that for psychiatric patients with other disorders ($n = 32$; 74.9 bpm).

Traumatic Stress

In a recent prospective study, Shalev and colleagues (1998b) examined the relationship between heart rate and blood pressure recorded immediately after a traumatic event and the development of PTSD 4 months later. Heart rate and blood pressure of 86 trauma survivors were recorded upon admission to an emergency room (ER) following trauma and then 1 week later. Subjects who had developed PTSD ($n = 20$) were compared with those who had not. As shown in Figure 7–1, both groups had elevated heart rate at the ER, yet the PTSD subjects, compared with the control subjects, had higher heart rate levels at the ER (95.5 ± 13.9 vs. 83.3 ± 10.9 bpm; $P < 0.001$) and 1 week later (77.8 ± 11.9 vs. 72.0 ± 9.5 bpm; $t = 2.25$, $P < 0.03$). The groups did not differ in initial blood pressure. The differences in heart rate between the two groups remained statistically significant when the intensity of the traumatic event, the intensity of the immediate response, and the effects of age and education were controlled and did not predict depression (Shalev et al. 1998a). Clinically, however, these differences may be of limited value because they overlap across groups.

Response to Challenge

Physical Exercise

Three years after the Lebanon War, we compared 48 combat veterans with PTSD with 50 combat veterans without PTSD on mea-

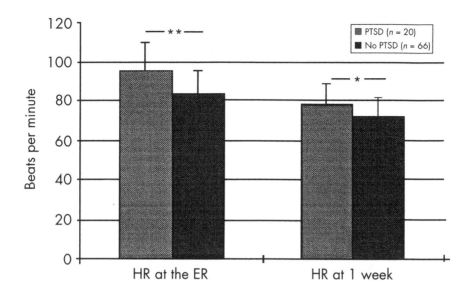

Figure 7–1. Heart rate (HR) levels in trauma survivors immediately after the trauma (in the emergency room [ER]) and 1 week later. The sample was divided into two groups based on presence of posttraumatic stress disorder (PTSD) at 4-month follow-up. *$P < 0.05$. **$P < 0.01$.

sures of effort tolerance (Shalev et al. 1990). Effort tolerance was evaluated by treadmill exercise, and the outcome measure was heart rate relative to degree of effort, body surface, and age. The results were expressed in percentage of the expected capacity for age/weight (PWC). PTSD patients had significantly lower PWC than control subjects (i.e., responded with higher heart rate to similar physical demands), and this effect was even greater when nonsmoking PTSD patients were compared with nonsmoking control subjects (73.3% for PTSD patients and 90% for control subjects). Moreover, eight PTSD patients could not complete the exercise because of what looked like an anxiety response (though a formal diagnosis of panic attack was not made).

Chemical Challenge

Two experiments, although only indirectly related to psychophysiology, are relevant to our discussion because they illustrate the general pattern of heightened responsivity in PTSD. Lactate infusion, which induces panic attacks in panic disorder patients, was found to provoke panic attacks and flashbacks in PTSD patients but not in control subjects (Reiman et al. 1989). In another study, yohimbine, an α_2-adrenergic receptor antagonist that activates brain norepinephrine activity, produced panic attacks in 70% and flashbacks in 40% of PTSD patients (Southwick et al. 1993).

Trauma-Related Cues

External Cues

Studies of physiological responses to cues reminiscent of the trauma (e.g., combat sounds) have consistently demonstrated that subjects with PTSD show a significant rise in heart rate, skin conduction, and blood pressure. The results from these studies are concordant across traumatized populations and experimental conditions and have been extensively reviewed (see Orr 1990; Prins et al. 1995; Shalev and Rogel-Fuchs 1993). Although clearly demonstrating a link between a cue reminiscent of the trauma and a physiological response, this methodological approach has not been used in a clinical setting, nor is there any way to test such responses prior to the traumatic event.

Mental Imagery of Traumatic Events

Several well-controlled studies (e.g., Pitman et al. 1987, 1990; Shalev et al. 1992b) have shown that combat veterans and civilians with PTSD, in response to making a mental image of their traumatic events, show markedly higher heart rate, skin conduction, and facial muscle activity (as assessed by the electromyogram [EMG]). In most of the studies, PTSD subjects did not show higher responses during mental imagery of other stressful events. In contrast, Shalev and colleagues (1992b) demonstrated elevated physiological responses to reminders of prior traumatizations in four civilian PTSD patients.

Mental Imagery of Nontraumatic Events

To further assess putative "reactivity" across stressful conditions, we explored the physiological responses of PTSD patients to imagery of a stressful event that preceded the onset of their illness but was not related to its cause. We used the the SCUD missile alarm during the Gulf War as the stressor, since experience of such an alarm was shared by all subjects (Shalev et al. 1996).

A mental imagery technique was used, in which a 30-second recording of the Gulf War missile alarm was presented to 12 PTSD patients, 11 panic disorder patients, 9 survivors of traumatic events who had not developed PTSD, and 19 psychiatrically healthy subjects with no history of major trauma. The PTSD group showed higher skin conduction and EMG responses to the Gulf War alarm (Figure 7–2), and the differences between the PTSD group and the

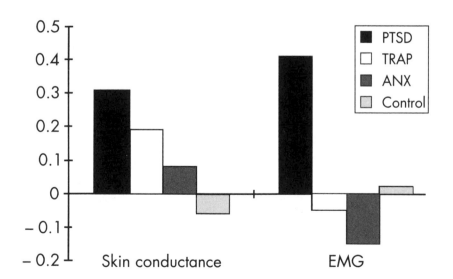

Figure 7–2. Physiological responses to Gulf War missile alarm presented in PTSD patients (n = 12), survivors of traumatic events who had not developed PTSD (n = 9) (TRAP), patients with anxiety disorders other than PTSD (n = 11) (ANX), and psychiatrically healthy subjects with no history of major trauma (n = 19) (Control). EMG = electromyogram.

other groups remained significant when age, levels of distress during the war, and concurrent anxiety were controlled. We tentatively concluded that patients with PTSD acquire and maintain prolonged physiological responses to several stressors during their life span. Alternatively, it can be argued that PTSD patients become sensitized to reminders of past traumas after the onset of their illness (a process also known as "reinstatement").

Mental Imagery in Recent Survivors

A potential use of the aforementioned mental imagery technique in the assessment of those at risk to develop PTSD is to identify, soon after the trauma, survivors who have an intense physiological response to recall of the trauma. To evaluate this effect, we studied responses to mental imagery of the trauma in 185 trauma survivors 4 months after the traumatic events. PTSD was diagnosed in 39 survivors (21%), and this group of subjects had significantly higher heart rate and frontalis EMG responses during mental imagery of their traumatic events when compared with the other survivors (Figure 7–3). As was stated above, the presence of elevated physiological responses to repeated recollections of a traumatic event can explain the progressive neuronal sensitization that may underlie PTSD.

Auditory Startle in Patients With PTSD

Exaggerated startle, one of the symptoms of increased arousal listed in the DSM-IV diagnostic criteria for PTSD (American Psychiatric Association 1994), has been reported in 86% of trauma survivors with PTSD (Davidson et al. 1991). Reports of exaggerated startle soon after exposure to trauma may have higher specificity for PTSD than do reports of intrusive imagery (McFarlane 1989).

In contrast, elevated eyeblink response has not been consistently found in PTSD, with three studies showing increased eyeblink EMG (Butler et al. 1990; Orr et al. 1995; Shalev et al. 1998b), and four others not finding such an elevation (Morgan et al. 1995; Orr et al. 1997; Ross et al. 1989; Shalev et al. 1992a). Studies of the auto-

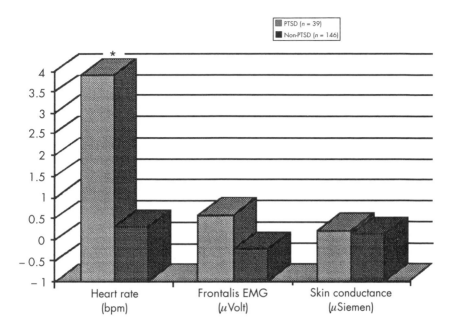

Figure 7–3. Response to mental imagery in 185 trauma survivors 4 months after the traumatic events. The sample was divided into two groups based on presence of posttraumatic stress disorder (PTSD) at 4-month follow-up. bpm = beats per minute. EMG = electromyogram. *Difference between groups significant at $P < 0.05$.

nomic component of the response (Orr et al. 1995, 1997; Paige et al. 1990; Shalev et al. 1992a, 1998b), however, consistently demonstrate an increased response and slower skin conductance habituation among PTSD patients.

Auditory Startle in Recent Trauma Survivors

Two lines of evidence suggested that the autonomic response to startle could signal a risk factor for PTSD. First, Lykken and colleagues (1988) showed that skin conductance habituation in psychiatrically healthy individuals is genetically determined. Second, Ohman and Bohlin (1973) demonstrated a positive correlation between skin conductance habituation and conditionability. On the basis of these studies, we hypothesized that impaired skin conductance habituation could preexist the trauma, predict the strong conditioning that leads to PTSD, and be detectable shortly after trauma in those who eventually develop PTSD (Shalev and Rogel-Fuchs 1993). However, this hypothesis has not been confirmed. In a prospective study of 218 trauma survivors, startle responses recorded 1 week after the trauma did not differentiate those who developed PTSD ($n = 37$) from those who did not. Rather, we found a progressive development of slow skin conductance habituation and elevated heart rate responses, occurring between 1 week and 4 months after trauma, in subjects who develop PTSD. These results can therefore be interpreted as defining a critical period during which the abnormalities that typically accompany chronic PTSD develop soon after the trauma (A. Y. Shalev, R. K. Pitman, S. P. Orr, et al., "Prospective Study of Responses to Loud Tones in Trauma Survivors With PTSD," submitted for publication, August 1988).

Startle Response During War Stress

To evaluate the effect of stressful events on auditory startle responses, we tested 10 healthy individuals 4 months before the Gulf War, during a missile alert on the first day of the war, and 8 months after the war (Shalev et al. 1996). The magnitude and the rate of habituation of orbicularis oculi EMG, heart rate, and skin conductance responses to 15 consecutive presentations of pure tones (95 dB, 0 rise time, 1,000 Hz) were recorded on each occasion, along with self-reports of anxiety.

The group's anxiety scores were significantly higher during the war, but the average auditory startle responses remained stable across exposure conditions. However, a notable decrease in skin conductance habituation was observed in two individuals who had been exposed to combat prior to the current stressor.

Such differences may illustrate a distinctive vulnerability to stress, since decreased autonomic habituation signals a decrease in the subject's capacity to correctly classify redundant and inconsequential stimulation (the repeated tones) as nonthreatening and to decrease his or her autonomic response appropriately. It is possible, therefore, that repeated exposure to extreme stress progressively erodes the individual's capacity to properly identify and respond to additional stressors. Such a trait is measurable in survivors of repeated traumatizations who have not developed PTSD and could be particularly valuable in evaluating parameters of attrition and stimulus discrimination in professionals whose work involves repeated exposure to major stressors.

Acquisition of Conditioned Responses

Using a differential aversive conditioning paradigm, Peri and colleagues (1994) experimentally elicited conditioned skin conductance responses by exposing PTSD patients and control subjects (who had been exposed to trauma in the past but had not developed PTSD) to neutral stimuli (colored lights), one of which was paired with loud noise. Peri et al. subsequently measured the magnitude, generalization, and extinction of the acquired autonomic responses. They found that PTSD subjects' skin conductance responses during acquisition were more intense than those of the control subjects. They also found that these responses, once acquired, extinguished less well in the PTSD patients and generalized to color slides that were not paired with noise. Peri et al. interpreted these results as suggesting that heightened conditionability or defaulted extinction plays a central role in the acquisition, maintenance, and overgeneralization of fear and avoidance in PTSD.

Conclusion

Several important factors related to the etiology of PTSD have been explored by psychophysiological studies. Data presented in this chapter show a consistent pattern of reactivity in PTSD. Data on heart rate at the time of traumatization suggest that such reactivity may precede the onset of PTSD. Heightened reactivity may reflect a biological endowment, prior learning, or concurrent appraisal and may be mediated by stress hormones such as cortisol or epinephrine. These parameters should be explored in future studies.

Peri et al.'s (1994) study of conditioning in PTSD and Shalev et al.'s (1997) study of responses to stressors that precede the trauma suggest that PTSD is associated with heightened conditionability and/or impaired extinction. Individual cases studied during the Gulf War further suggest that problems in stimulus discrimination may result from prior exposure to traumatic stress and affect the responses to subsequent events. Finally, the prospective study of auditory startle in PTSD (Shalev et al. 1998b) has tentatively outlined a critical period during which the neurobiological processes that lead to PTSD are operating.

The final word, however, is one of caution for several reasons: First, the current data do not allow us to clearly differentiate expressions related to the causes of PTSD ("risk factors") from those that are related to the presence of the disorder. Second, the relative contribution of any risk factor must be evaluated in the context of the total causation, and redundancy with other factors is to be expected. Hence, the data presented in this chapter should be considered as suggestive and as opening the way for further studies.

References

American Psychiatric Association: Diagnostic and Statistical Manual of Mental Disorders, 4th Edition. Washington, DC, American Psychiatric Association, 1994

Bateson P: The interpretation of sensitive periods, in The Behavior of Human Infants, Edited by Olivero, Zapella. New York, Plenum, 1984, pp 57–70

Baum A: Stress, intrusive imagery, and chronic distress. Health Psychol 9:653–675, 1990

Breslau N, Davis GC: Posttraumatic stress disorder in an urban population of young adults: risk factors for chronicity. Am J Psychiatry 149: 671–675, 1992

Butler RW, Braff DL, Rausch JL, et al: Physiological evidence of exaggerated startle response in a subgroup of Vietnam veterans with combat-related PTSD. Am J Psychiatry 147:1308–1312, 1990

Charney DS, Deutch AY, Krystal JH, et al: Psychobiologic mechanisms of posttraumatic stress disorder. Arch Gen Psychiatry 50:295–305, 1993

Davidson JRT, Hughes D, Blazer D, et al: Posttraumatic stress disorder in the community: an epidemiological study. Psychol Med 21:1–9, 1991

Davis M, Walker DL, Lee Y: Roles of the amygdala and bed nucleus of the stria terminalis in fear and anxiety measured with the acoustic startle reflex: possible relevance to PTSD. Ann N Y Acad Sci 821:305–331, 1997

Gerardi RJ, Keane TM, Cahoon BJ, et al: An in vivo assessment of physiological arousal in posttraumatic stress disorder. J Abnorm Psychol 103:825–827, 1994

Keane TM, Fairbank JA, Caddel MT, et al: A behavioral approach to assessing and treating post-traumatic stress disorders in Vietnam veterans, in Trauma and Its Wake: The Study and Treatment of Post-Traumatic Stress Disorder. Edited by Figley CR. New York, Brunner/Mazel, 1985, pp 257–294

Kolb LC: A neuropsychological hypothesis explaining the post-traumatic stress disorder. Am J Psychiatry 144:989–999, 1987

Lykken DT, Iacono KH, Haroian K, et al: Habituation of the skin conductance response to strong stimuli: a twin study. Psychophysiology 25:4–15, 1988

McFall ME, Murburg MM: Psychophysiological studies of combat-related PTSD: an integrated view, in Catecholamine Function in Post-traumatic Stress Disorder: Emerging Concepts. Edited by Murburg MM. Washington, DC, American Psychiatric Press, 1994, pp 161–173

McFall ME, Veith RC, Murburg MM: Basal sympathoadrenal function in PTSD. Biol Psychiatry 31:1050–1056, 1992

McFarlane AC: The phenomenology of post-traumatic stress disorder following a natural disaster. J Nerv Ment Dis 176:22–29, 1989

Morgan CA III, Grillon C, Southwick SM, et al: Fear-potentiated startle in post-traumatic stress disorder. Biol Psychiatry 38:378–385, 1995

Morgan CA III, Grillon C, Southwick SM, et al: Exaggerated acoustic startle reflex in Gulf War veteran with PTSD. Am J Psychiatry 153:64–68, 1996

North CS, Smith EM: Posttraumatic stress disorder among homeless men and women. Hospital and Community Psychiatry 43:1010–1016, 1992

Ohman A, Bohlin G. Magnitude and habituation of the orienting reaction as predictors of discriminative electrodermal conditioning. Journal of Experimental Research in Personality 6:293–299, 1973

Orr SP: Psychophysiological studies of PTSD, in Biological Assessment and Treatment of Posttraumatic Stress Disorder. Edited by Giller E. Washington, DC, American Psychiatric Press, 1990, pp 137–157

Orr SP, Lasko N, Shalev A, et al: Physiologic responses to loud tone in Vietnam veterans with PTSD. J Abnorm Psychol 104:75–82, 1995

Orr SP, Solomon Z, Peri T, et al: Physiological responses to loud tone in Israeli war veterans of the 1973 Yom Kippur War. Biol Psychiatry 41:319–326, 1997

Paige SR, Graham M, Reid MG, et al: Psychophysiological correlates of posttraumatic stress disorder in Vietnam veterans. Biol Psychiatry 27:419–430, 1990

Peri T. Ben-Shachar G, Shalev A: Heightened conditionability in PTSD and panic disorder. Paper presented at the 147th annual meeting of the American Psychiatric Association, Philadelphia, May 1994

Pitman RK, Orr SP, Forgue DF, et al: Psychophysiology of PTSD imagery in Vietnam combat veterans. Arch Gen Psychiatry 44:970–975, 1987

Pitman RK, Orr SP, Forgue DF, et al: Psychophysiologic responses to combat imagery of Vietnam veterans with post-traumatic stress disorder versus other anxiety disorders. J Abnorm Psychol 99:49–54, 1990

Prins A, Kaloupek DG, Keane TM: Psychophysiological evidence for autonomic arousal and startle in PTSD, in Neurobiological and Clinical Consequences of Stress. Edited by Friedman JM, Charney DS, Deutch AY. Philadelphia, PA, JB Lippincott–Raven, 1995, pp 291–314

Reiman EM, Raichele ME, Robins E, et al: Neuroanatomical correlates of lactate-induced anxiety attack. Arch Gen Psychiatry 46:493–500, 1989

Ross RJ, Ball WA, Cohen ME, et al: Habituation of the startle reflex in posttraumatic stress disorder. J Neuropsychiatry Clin Neurosci 1:305–307, 1989

Shalev AY, Rogel-Fuchs Y: Psychophysiology of the post-traumatic stress disorder: from sulfur fumes to behavioral genetics. Psychosom Med 55:413–423, 1993

Shalev AY, Bleich A, Ursano RJ: Posttraumatic stress disorder: somatic comorbidity and effort symptoms. Psychosomatics 31:197–203, 1990

Shalev AY, Orr SP, Peri T, et al: Physiologic responses to loud tones in Israeli patients with posttraumatic stress disorder. Arch Gen Psychiatry 49:870–875, 1992a

Shalev AY, Orr SP, Pitman RK: Psychophysiologic response during script driven imagery as an outcome measure in post-traumatic stress disorder. J Clin Psychiatry 53:324–326, 1992b

Shalev AY, Peri T, Bonne O: Auditory startle response during exposure to war stress. Compr Psychiatry 37:134–138, 1996

Shalev AY, Peri T, Gelpin E, et al: Psychophysiologic assessment of mental imagery of stressful events in Israeli civilian PTSD patients. Compr Psychiatry 38:269–273, 1997

Shalev AY, Freedman S, Peri T, et al: Prospective study of posttraumatic stress disorder and depression following trauma. Am J Psychiatry 155:630–637, 1998a

Shalev AY, Sahar T, Freedman S, et al: A prospective study of heart rate responses following trauma and the subsequent development of PTSD. Arch Gen Psychiatry 55:553–559, 1998b

Southwick SM, Krystal JH, Morgan CA, et al: Abnormal noradrenergic function in posttraumatic stress disorder. Arch Gen Psychiatry 50: 266–274, 1993

True WR, Rice J, Eisen SA, et al: A twin study of genetic and environmental contributions to liability for posttraumatic stress symptoms. Arch Gen Psychiatry 50:257–264, 1993

Zeitlin SB, McNally RJ: Implicit and explicit memory bias for threat in post-traumatic stress disorder. Behav Res Ther 29:451–457, 1991

Chapter 8

Risk Factors for the Acute Biological and Psychological Response to Trauma

A. C. McFarlane, M.D., F.R.A.N.Z.C.P., M.B.B.S.
(Dip.Psychother.)

The relationship between the acute biological and psychological response to trauma is a key theoretical issue in understanding posttraumatic stress disorder (PTSD). The central underlying question is the extent to which the reaction of the individual at the time of the traumatic event is related to the psychopathology and neurobiology of any disorder that emerges. The initial hypothesis, formulated at the turn of the 20th century, proposed that in PTSD there was an exaggerated response at the time of the traumatic event (van der Kolk et al. 1996). This formulation, in part, arose from notions about the relation of cowardice and uncontrolled fear at the time of the trauma to subsequent psychopathology. A legacy of this hypothesis, when PTSD was first included in the DSM classification (in DSM-III [American Psychiatric Association 1980]), was that the neurobiology of PTSD was, in effect, the neurobiology of stress.

However, it has been increasingly recognized over the past two decades that the relationships among PTSD, the stressor, and its acute effects are somewhat more complex (Yehuda and McFarlane 1995). First, any description of these relationships needs to take into account the fact that the majority of individuals who experience trauma, even the most extreme trauma, do not develop PTSD. Thus, in only a minority of people will there be a progression to the disorder. Second, as this book attests, the existence of risk factors other than the trauma as predictors of PTSD highlights the interactional nature of the etiological process. This disorder, in other words, is not a normal response to an abnormal experience. Third, the prevalence of posttraumatic comorbidity does not confirm the uniqueness or independence of PTSD after exposure to trauma. PTSD is only one of a number of disorders that emerge in this context, further implying the role of a matrix of risk factors that determine these differential outcomes.

The role of risk factors can be mediated at various points in an etiological pathway (Figure 8–1). Hence, there is a need to investigate the difference between the stress response in those who develop PTSD with a chronic course and the response in those whose PTSD symptoms are relatively short lived. Furthermore, risk factors may influence the consolidation and remission of symptoms. In particular, data from a variety of sources suggest that factors influencing the immediate recovery period may play a central role in the development of the disorder (McFarlane 1989). The data further suggest that this may be a period during which critical neurobiological alterations occur. In this chapter, I examine some of the possible risk factors that exert their influence during this critical period and operate by influencing the magnitude and type of the acute trauma response.

The question of to what extent the acute reaction to the traumatic event is related to subsequent psychopathology is not a new one

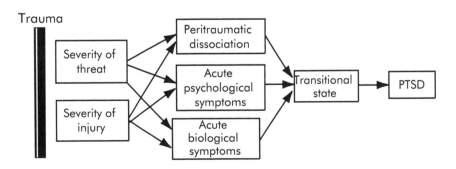

Figure 8–1. Possible pathway for the impact of risk factors in acute stress reaction. PTSD = posttraumatic stress disorder.

and has long influenced the formulations of the psychopathology of trauma. The historical views that have influenced the investigation of this question are outlined in the sections that follow. Critical to understanding this relationship is the conceptual issue of the nature of the relationship between the acute distress and subsequent psychopathology. The transitional nature of this etiological process and the role of risk factors in this progression are highlighted in this chapter. To date, there are limited empirical data on the relationship between the acute stress response and emerging psychopathological syndromes.

The neurobiological systems and psychological processes that form the foundations of the acute stress response provide important insights into the systems and processes. These systems form the springboard from which psychopathological syndromes that arise in response to trauma emerge. This conceptualization suggests that the nature of the disorder can be understood by examining the possible disruptions that occur in these regulatory systems of memory and arousal. However, at this stage, we have limited knowledge about the differences between the normal and maladaptive reactions of these systems. One of the problems is that many of the animal models of research that have been used to develop hypotheses about the stress response in general are not applicable to the traumatic stress response in humans.

In this chapter, I do not address the impact of different types of traumatic experience or their subcomponents as risk factors, despite the relevance of such issues to an understanding of the nature of acute stress disorders. Traumatic stressors vary along a variety of dimensions, such as duration, severity of the threat to life, extent of injury, and loss of life and property (McFarlane and de Girolamo 1996). Although the nature of the experience may have an impact on the pattern of acute distress and, hence, may influence the risk factors that may be brought into play, there is little prospective research to draw on, and so the area will not be discussed (Weisaeth 1996). However, it will suffice to indicate that Breslau and colleagues (1991) suggested that the type of traumatic experience may have a major impact on the long-term course of PTSD. Somewhat surprisingly, brief and circumscribed traumas such as accidents may have more enduring effects than combat (Norris 1992). However, the small numbers and limited range of traumas documented in these two studies limit the capacity to generalize from their findings. These findings indicate the need to look at whether the risk factors described in this chapter may have elements that are specific to particular classes of traumatic events.

Furthermore, many other factors, such as prior experience, training, the immediate social environment, the behavior of others, adequacy of rescue, and leadership, have a substantial capacity to modulate traumatic experiences (Weisaeth 1996). Although the role of these factors has been commented on extensively, there is, again, little systematic research that has linked them to the acute outcomes and, secondarily, to PTSD. The uncertainty in this area of knowledge is reflected in the apparently contradictory evidence about the benefits of single-session debriefing in close proximity to an event that may worsen outcome rather than lead to improvement as the many anecdotal reports would suggest (Raphael et al. 1996).

In discussing the acute role of risk factors, it is first necessary to review the current conceptualization of acute stress disorders and their role as risk factors for chronic PTSD.

Current Conceptualization of Acute Stress Disorders

The inadequacy of the research data on the nature of the relationship between trauma and subsequent psychopathology arises because very few of the many studies of traumatic stress have focused on describing or investigating the cause of the range of immediate reactions. This is in part because war and disasters are very difficult times in which to conduct research. It was only in DSM-IV (American Psychiatric Association 1994) that a diagnosis to describe the acute reactions to severe traumatic events was formulated (Table 8–1). DSM-IV emphasizes the presence of acute dissociative reactions in combination with PTSD that emerge at the time of exposure to the event, as described by Spiegel (1991, 1997) in his influential work. In part, these criteria reflect the role of acute

Table 8–1. DSM-IV diagnostic criteria for acute stress disorder

A. The person has been exposed to a traumatic event in which both of the following were present:

 (1) the person experienced, witnessed, or was confronted with an event or events that involved actual or threatened death or serious injury, or a threat to the physical integrity of self or others
 (2) the person's response involved intense fear, helplessness, or horror

B. Either while experiencing or after experiencing the distressing event, the individual has three (or more) of the following dissociative symptoms:

 (1) a subjective sense of numbing, detachment, or absence of emotional responsiveness
 (2) a reduction in awareness of his or her surroundings (e.g., "being in a daze")
 (3) derealization
 (4) depersonalization
 (5) dissociative amnesia (i.e., inability to recall an important aspect of the trauma)

C. The traumatic event is persistently reexperienced in at least one of the following ways: recurrent images, thoughts, dreams, illusions, flashback episodes, or a sense of reliving the experience; or distress on exposure to reminders of the traumatic event.

D. Marked avoidance of stimuli that arouse recollections of the trauma (e.g., thoughts, feelings, conversations, activities, places, people).

E. Marked symptoms of anxiety or increased arousal (e.g., difficulty sleeping, irritability, poor concentration, hypervigilance, exaggerated startle response, motor restlessness).

F. The disturbance causes clinically significant distress or impairment in social, occupational, or other important areas of functioning or impairs the individual's ability to pursue some necessary task, such as obtaining necessary assistance or mobilizing personal resources by telling family members about the traumatic experience.

(continued)

Table 8–1. DSM-IV diagnostic criteria for acute stress disorder
(*continued*)

G. The disturbance lasts for a minimum of 2 days and a maximum of 4 weeks and occurs within 4 weeks of the traumatic event.

H. The disturbance is not due to the direct physiological effects of a substance (e.g., a drug of abuse, a medication) or a general medical condition, is not better accounted for by Brief Psychotic Disorder, and is not merely an exacerbation of a preexisting Axis I or Axis II disorder.

Source.   Reprinted from American Psychiatric Association: *Diagnostic and Statistical Manual of Mental Disorders,* 4th Edition. Washington, DC, American Psychiatric Press, 1994. Copyright 1994, American Psychiatric Association. Used with permission.

dissociation as a critical component of long-term posttraumatic reactions. In contrast, the ICD-10 (World Health Organization 1992) definition is more reflective of the descriptions that have been accumulated from military psychiatry and are perhaps more specific to combat. This definition focuses on the polymorphic nature of the symptoms and the rapidly fluctuating phenomenology, and anxiety, depression, and lability are given more emphasis.

These criteria sets will have an important impact on the investigation of the nature and the prevalence of acute stress reactions in the same way that the DSM-III diagnostic criteria for PTSD provided a benchmark for the development of the investigation of chronic traumatic reactions. These definitions have a particularly potent capacity to focus investigations into the exact nature of the acute stress reactions that are especially detrimental to long-term adaptation and their relationship to the psychophysiology and biochemistry of the normal stress response.

Historical Formulation

The hypothesis of the importance of the pattern of reaction at the time of the traumatic event is a central feature of the early formulations about the pathogenic potential of traumatic events. This pattern, according to these early formulations, creates a state of mind that then molds the individual's long-term psychopathology. The implication is that the event becomes embedded in the mind of the individual, reorganizing his or her subsequent affect regulation and cognition.

Breuer and Freud (1893–1895/1955) believed that traumatic experiences have two primary characteristics. The person experiences an intense state of fear during which he or she is unable to react, and from these experiences arise dissociative states that prevent the integration of the experience. Breuer and Freud believed that the potential to develop these hypnoid states has a characterological dimension. Janet (1909) emphasized the centrality of the interaction of affect and memory. It was his view that "[f]orgetting the event which precipitated the emotion . . . has frequently been found to accompany intense emotional experiences in the form of continuous and retrograde amnesia" (p. 1607). He claimed that a person is "unable to make the recital which we call narrative memory, and yet he remains confronted by [the] difficult situation" (Janet 1925, p. 660). This results in "a phobia of memory" (Janet, 1925, p. 661) that prevents the integration ("synthesis") of traumatic events and splits off the traumatic memories from ordinary consciousness. Thus, Breuer and Freud and Janet proposed that intense arousal interferes with proper information processing and with appropriate action and that because of such interference the storage of information into narrative (explicit) memory is disrupted.

These early views strongly influenced the view in World War I that a soldier's behavior on the battlefield was the critical determinant of "shell shock" or "traumatic neurosis" (Leed 1979). Given the intensity of trench warfare and the failure of military tactics and morale in the face of the extraordinary casualties, it is easy to see how concepts of cowardice and bravery could become confused with acute stress disorders. This further added a pejorative assessment of those who developed these disorders without any evidence of maladaptive behavior at the time of battle.

The extent to which particular "peri-traumatic" reactions (e.g.,

dissociation, freezing–surrender, disorganization) specifically predict prolonged distress was more systematically examined in
World War II. Grinker and Spiegel (1945) proposed that some people develop excessive responses under stress and that such responses are often transformed into prolonged disorders.

> Fear and anger in small doses are stimulating and alert the ego, in-
> creasing efficacy. But, when stimulated by repeated psychological
> trauma[,] the intensity of the emotion heightens until a point is
> reached at which the ego loses its effectiveness and may become al-
> together crippled. . . . The clinical description of the neurotic reac-
> tions to severe combat stress is thus a passing parade of every type
> of psychological and psychosomatic symptom, and of maladaptive
> behavior. In addition[,] one of the major characteristics of traits of
> neurotic reactions to battle is the manner in which symptoms alter
> with the lapse of time. (p. 82)

Grinker and Spiegel (1954) also proposed a hierarchy of combat
anxiety states:

> [M]ild anxiety states in which the subjective and motor signs of anx-
> iety are present but function is not yet interfered with. In moderate
> anxiety states the same symptoms may have progressed to the point
> where the flier makes mistakes in flying and now has his own inca-
> pacity to fear as well. . . . Severe anxiety states . . . [entail] much re-
> gression of the ego, confusion in regard to the environment, mutism
> and stupor. (p. 84)

These historical formulations provide a set of hypotheses
around which to examine the role of various risk factors in the
emergence of PTSD from the acute stress response.

Acute Stress Disorder as a Risk Factor for PTSD

The relationship between acute stress disorders and chronic PTSD
has been examined more systematically in Israeli war veterans by
Solomon and colleagues (1996). In general, in some cases the
pathogenic effects of acute stress disorders may abate, whereas in

others there may be profound, prolonged, and varied psychological sequelae.

Solomon and Kleinhauz (1996) showed that PTSD occurs with much greater frequency among soldiers with acute stress disorders than among other combat-exposed soldiers. They also found that the prognosis for spontaneous recovery is significantly better in those who do not have an acute stress disorder (37% of acute stress disorder casualties who reported having PTSD in the past still had the syndrome at the time of the study, compared with 23% of the control group). Not all combat stress reaction casualties experience long-term maladjustment, however; this study also showed a substantial pattern of recovery over time.

The link between acute stress disorder and PTSD may result from several sources. Soldiers who develop acute combat stress reactions experience a wide range of distress and non-PTSD psychiatric symptoms (Solomon 1989, 1993), a finding which emphasizes that PTSD is only one of a range of posttraumatic adaptations. Combat stress may also have long-lasting effects on the social aspects of the veteran's life (DeFazio et al. 1975; Figley 1978). Combat stress–related casualties reported more problems in work performance, family functioning, sexual functioning, and various aspects of social functioning than did control subjects (Solomon 1993). The difficulties in most of these areas did not abate with time. Only problems in family functioning were reported by fewer soldiers 3 years after the war than at the end of the first year (Solomon 1994). A higher proportion of individuals who were combat stress–related casualties, relative to control subjects, reported higher rates of somatic complaints and behaviors potentially detrimental to their health (Solomon 1988; Solomon and Mikulincer 1987; Solomon et al. 1987). In general, individuals who were combat stress–related casualties reported poorer health than did control subjects (Solomon 1994).

Dissociation and Acute Symptoms as Risk Factors

The role of a variety of psychological symptoms as potential risk factors has not been extensively investigated. Apart from the Israeli armed forces studies (Solomon 1993), Rachman's (1990) study of the Blitz in London, and Saigh's (1984) study of students in Beirut, very little systematic research has been done in war. Studies of the acute reactions to other traumatic events include those of the victims of terrorist bombings (Shalev 1992), a factory explosion (Weisaeth 1989a, 1989b), and motor vehicle accidents (Barton et al. 1996; Malt et al. 1989; Mayou et al. 1993). Though few in number, these studies are critical, since most of the observations about the acute antecedents of PTSD have been developed in retrospective clinical observation of patients and are in need of refinement in the light of prospective studies. Prospective studies suggest that the dynamic interrelationships among intrusion, avoidance, and arousal may be somewhat different in the acute, and much more unstable, phase of reaction than 1 month after the traumatic experience.

The 1980s produced research examining the nature of early posttraumatic reactions in populations exposed to disaster. These populations were generally identified in relatively close proximity to the event, and in many cases follow-up was conducted. This research led to the reformulation, in DSM-IV, that the experiences of helplessness and powerlessness were central aspects of the acute response to the traumatic event if the individual was going to develop PTSD. This is in contrast to the stressor criterion of DSM-III, which focused only on the quality of the event. This reformulation was in part encouraged by the reemergence of an interest in dissociation as one of the main components of the phenomenology of PTSD (Atchison and McFarlane 1994).

The role of dissociation has been investigated empirically by several groups of researchers, who concluded that the occurrence of dissociation during the time of the trauma predicts development of PTSD (Holen 1990; Spiegel 1991). Other groups of researchers (Bremner et al. 1995; Marmar et al. 1994) looked at this issue in Vietnam War veterans. These latter studies, however, were conducted more than 20 years after exposure to the trauma, and this raises some important questions as to whether the symptoms of the disorder may modify the retrospective recall of the nature of the traumatic experience. Several studies (Koopman et al. 1994; Shalev

et al. 1996; Weiss et al. 1995) investigated this issue in closer proximity to the event and again highlighted the importance of
peritraumatic dissociation. Shalev and co-workers' report was particularly noteworthy because the subjects were studied within
2 weeks of the accident. However, Malt and colleagues (Malt and
Olafsen 1992; Malt et al. 1989), in a study of accident victims who
were interviewed during hospital admission, did not confirm this
finding. In fact, Lundin (1996) found that peritraumatic dissociation protected people from the subsequent onset of psychiatric
morbidity.

A recently completed study examined the acute patterns of reaction within 24 hours of subjects' being admitted to hospital after
motor vehicle accidents and how these patterns predicted subsequent depression and PTSD (McFarlane 1997). Twenty-four hours
postaccident, the subjects who subsequently developed PTSD or
major depression could not be differentiated from the subjects who
did not develop any psychiatric disorder on the basis of the nature
of their symptomatic reactions (e.g., intrusions, avoidance, hyperarousal, and dissociation). Ten days after the accident, however, it
was beginning to be possible to differentiate the groups on the
basis of each of these symptoms. These findings are similar to those
of Weisaeth (1989a), who demonstrated that failure of anxiety
symptoms to remit in the first 2 weeks was a significant risk factor
for PTSD. However, Shalev (1992) found that acute symptoms of
intrusion and anxiety had little predictive ability for PTSD among
the victims of a terrorist bombing. This raises the interesting question as to whether any particular component of the acute reaction
is the core of the reaction that drives the other components and
hence represents the primary risk factor. In the more established
stage of PTSD, it appears that intrusion plays the primary role in
mediating between arousal and the traumatic experience (McFarlane 1992).

McFarlane and colleagues (1997) have noted the complexity of
determining the role of dissociation. Dissociation should not be
seen simply as an independent variable that describes the nature of
the individual's reaction at the time of the event. Dissociative
symptoms are found to be more prevalent in those with a family

history of psychiatric disorder or a past history of psychiatric disorder. Also, dissociative reaction at the time of the traumatic event can lead to the individual's behaving in a way that might increase his or her exposure to the traumatic incident because of an inability to behave in an adaptive way. One explanation for the suggestion in retrospective studies that peritraumatic dissociation is important as a predictor of long-term outcome involves the problem of accurate retrospective recall, which may be a factor even with studies that assess individuals at the time of the accident and at a later time in close proximity to the accident (7–10 days). Hence, the exact role of dissociation as a risk factor requires further elucidation.

A reexamination of Foa's (1997) treatment outcome data leads to some interesting observations about risk factors for chronicity of posttraumatic reactions. Foa found that if the most severe symptoms did not occur in the immediate aftermath of the trauma (i.e., delayed maximal intensity of symptoms), there was a greater risk of poor response to treatment. Anger at the time of the event decreased the severity of the acute symptoms, but it also tended to interfere with the effectiveness of treatment. The emergence of a high degree of distress when the patient recalled the traumatic experience, which suggests emotional engagement, predicted good outcome in a treatment setting. However, it remains to be tested whether these same phenomena predicted the emergence of chronic PTSD in settings where the individual is not receiving treatment.

Organization of Traumatic Memories as Early Risk Factors

Relatively little systematic research has been conducted on the relationship between the organization of traumatic memories and long-term outcome. van der Kolk and Fisler (1995) investigated this question using a traumatic memories inventory that measures the way in which traumatic experiences are retrieved. The process of recall of traumatic events was compared with that of personally significant nontraumatic events. Among those in the sample who had experienced trauma as children, it was demonstrated that narrative memory of the event was disrupted. Such disruption was also reported for 78% of the individuals who had experienced trauma as adults. Regardless of the age at which the trauma occurred, the memory of the trauma tended to occur initially in the form of somatosensory flashback experiences as visual, olfactory, affective, auditory, or somaesthetic imprints. The capacity to describe what had happened tended to emerge over time.

These data support the notion that traumatic memories are initially laid down in such a way that the sensory components are relatively fragmented and a more composite picture of the experience emerges with the passage of time. However, it remains to be investigated whether such fragmentation is a characteristic of the traumatic experience per se or whether the memory disturbance is more disrupted among individuals with PTSD and, therefore, an important risk factor in the immediate aftermath of an experience.

The structure of the traumatic narrative has also been investigated in treatment populations. Foa (1997) provided some important evidence of the deficiency of the narrative of the traumatic experience and demonstrated the way more complex descriptions of thoughts and feelings and more organizing thoughts emerge in the course of treatment. Tromp and colleagues (1995) showed that individuals with PTSD use more speech fillers, repetitions, and incomplete sentences. These individuals' description of the traumatic event had more disconnection of time and space, and the thought utterance reflected confusion. Future studies of the structure of the traumatic narrative need to be carried out in closer temporal proximity to the traumatic event, because time is one variable that could account for the progressive modification found among individuals with PTSD.

Peritraumatic Coping as a Predictor of Outcome

Different coping styles at the time of traumatic events have also been investigated as acute risk factors. Shalev and Munitz (1989) defined coping during combat as any attempt to increase the gap between combat stress and subjective distress, a definition that has general applicability. A variety of ways have been used to conceptualize coping, including problem-focused, emotion-focused, and appraisal-related approaches (e.g., Haan 1969; Lazarus and Folkman 1984). Solomon and colleagues (1990a, 1990b) and Spurrell and McFarlane (1995) found that the use of all coping strategies was associated with the presence of PTSD, an indication of the problem of retrospective bias in the interpretation of other studies. In contrast, Solomon et al. (1990a) found that emotion-focused coping and blunting coping strategies were associated with long-term psychiatric symptoms, whereas problem-focused coping and monitoring coping strategies moderated the detrimental effects of emotion-focused coping on mental health.

One possible explanation for the discrepancies between these findings is that the types of coping that optimize survival are different from those recruited in response to other life events. The available measures were derived from this more general field of research. Effective coping results in relief of personal distress, maintenance of a sense of personal worth, conservation of one's ability to form rewarding social contacts, and a sustained capability to meet the requirements of the task (Pearlin and Schooler 1978). Hence, passive surrender, stoic acceptance, and cognitive-reframing are appropriate in situations where the stressor is uncontrollable, whereas direct action on the stressor, help seeking, and other active coping strategies are adaptive in other circumstances. This complexity has not been addressed in the investigation of traumatic stressors to date.

In a study of survivors of a terrorist attack, Shalev (1992) described a wide variety of coping efforts during the impact phase of the stressor. These included actively rescuing other survivors, sharing important information with the rescuers, preserving one's dignity by covering one's body, and controlling the disclosure of information about the event to one's relatives. Even survivors who were severely injured seemed to have engaged in some mode of coping during and immediately after the event. The survivors described that successfully achieving their individual coping goals increased their sense of control and reduced their distress.

Acute Biological Risk Factors

A question of fundamental importance pertains to the nature of the acute biological stress response and its relationship to adverse traumatic outcomes, such as PTSD and major depressive disorder. Many of the formulations about the chronic neurobiology of PTSD are based on theoretical formulations as to how these chronic disturbances might relate to the nature of the acute response at the time of traumatic exposure. As has been described, conducting research on acutely traumatized individuals is highly problematic from both practical and ethical perspectives. For this reason, much of the data discussed is derived from animal models. However, it has not always been clear that the experimental conditions of stress in animal work are analagous to the stressors that produce PTSD in humans.

The biology of PTSD is different in many respects from that found in animal stress experiments (cf. Yehuda and Antelman 1993). Indeed, the lack of utility of such animal models is demonstrated by the observation that the biological alterations in PTSD are different from the normative responses to stress formulated by Selye (1956) in terms of variables such as the nature and persistence of the alterations. Furthermore, animal stress models seldom take into account intraspecies differences in reactivity to stress, an issue that is critical to understanding the role of risk factors in humans.

Hence, there is a fundamental interest in the way in which the acute biological stress response in individuals who go on to develop PTSD differs from that in individuals who develop major depression or no psychiatric disorder. The pattern of responsiveness of the hypothalamic-pituitary-adrenal (HPA) axis at the time of the trauma is an area of critical interest, given the importance of the abnormalities of this system that have been identified (see Chapter 1, this volume). In a small preliminary pilot investigation of accident survivors, McFarlane and colleagues (1997) found that serum cortisol levels from samples taken shortly after the trauma predicted outcome, whereas acute (day 1) psychological reactions did not. The cortisol sample was taken from blood drawn to measure the individual's blood alcohol immediately after the accident. This sample, taken on average 2 hours after the accident, found that the PTSD group had the lowest rise in cortisol levels and the group who later developed major depressive disorder the highest rise in cortisol levels. Thus, the acute neurobiological stress response apparently had some ability to predict the onset of psychiatric disorder 6 months later, in contrast to the acute psychological state.

A question that has not been answered is whether these HPA abnormalities arise from an abnormal HPA response at the time of the trauma or develop later in the course of the illness. Further understanding of HPA responses at the time of trauma in individuals who later develop PTSD may give insight into biological vulnerabilities and perhaps allow identification of "at risk" individuals. The body of literature concerning HPA abnormalities in PTSD has generally studied populations many years after the initial trauma, and this raises the strong possibility that intervening factors contributed to the HPA abnormalities. One small study assessed acute cortisol levels in rape victims (Resnick et al. 1995). Acute cortisol responses did not predict the development of PTSD, but those subjects with a history of prior trauma showed attenuated cortisol responses and were at greater risk of developing PTSD. These findings suggest that prior trauma may "sensitize" an individual's biological response to later trauma, leaving him or her at greater risk for PTSD. It should be noted, however, that this study included only 24 subjects, and a larger sample is needed before more definitive statements can be made. Also, factors affecting the acute stress response apart from prior trauma were not taken into account.

In PTSD, the role of cortisol in the acute stress response is of great interest because of the way cortisol may modulate the hormonal changes that in turn influence learning and memory, which are critical to understanding the etiology of PTSD. The suggestion has been made that traumatic events may cause an overstimulation of stress-activated neuropeptides such as adrenocorticotropic hormone (ACTH) and vasopressin, which in turn may result in an overconsolidation of memory (Southwick et al. 1994). It has been proposed that this overconsolidation of memory may lead to the intrusive recollections of PTSD. The modulatory or antistress effects of cortisol may therefore be essential to understanding PTSD. Essentially, if cortisol shuts off all the other biological reactions, such as the neuropeptide and catecholamine reactions, the inability to mount an effective cortisol response at the time of the trauma is likely to put an individual at risk for developing PTSD. In this regard, the implications of the finding that chronic PTSD is associated with low basal cortisol levels (Yehuda and McFarlane 1995) are of particular interest.

It is important to better characterize these acute responses in individuals who go on to develop PTSD because of the different implications of basal cortisol levels and cortisol levels at the time of the acute stress response. The HPA axis controls both tonic and phasic cortisol secretion, so it is possible that individuals could have low cortisol levels at baseline and still show a good stress response, and vice versa. Thus, the data on cortisol secretion in patients with chronic PTSD do not in any way inform us of what the individual's cortisol response was at the time of trauma. Therefore, Resnick et al.'s (1995) findings, in conjunction with pilot data conducted by McFarlane et al. (1997), are of particular importance, because they raise the possibility that the inability to mount an effective cortisol response at the time of a trauma might place the individual at particular risk for developing PTSD and that this inability cannot be assumed from the basal cortisol levels in chronic PTSD. Hence, this study, because of its theoretical importance, needs to be validated with a group of victims who have experienced a different type of trauma.

The acute stress response to trauma has also been studied in relation to heart rate. Shalev (1997), in a follow-up study, examined heart rate in 86 trauma survivors at the time of presentation to the emergency room (ER) of a hospital in Israel. Excluding subjects who had significant physical injury, the subjects who later developed PTSD had a higher heart rate in the ER at the time of evaluation (95.45 ± 13.9 vs. 83.44 ± 10.8 with posttraumatic symptoms [but no PTSD] and 83 ± 11.49 in individuals without PTSD) and at 1 week after the trauma, but not later. Even when a number of potential complicating factors, such as the intensity of the trauma, the nature of the immediate psychological stress response, and peritraumatic dissociation were examined, the difference in heart rate remained significant. The prospective nature of these data indicates the potential importance of the role of the sympathetic and parasympathetic nervous systems as risk factors in the acute stress response.

An elegant body of research demonstrates the role of norepinephrine in the acute stress response and the consolidation of emotional memory (Cahill 1997). Emotional arousal, correlated with activation of the right amygdala, has been shown to correlate with accuracy of recall (Cahill et al. 1995). This effect can be blocked with beta-adrenergic blockers. Although such studies have not been conducted for PTSD, theoretically these observations of Cahill may indicate that the pattern of catecholamine response at the time of the trauma may be critical in determining the signature of the traumatic memory. The modification of these memories in the immediate aftermath of the traumatic experience is also thought to be critical. Much evidence attests to the susceptibility of memory storage processes to modulating influences after learning provides the opportunity for emotional activation to regulate the strength of memory traces representing important experiences (Gold and McGaugh 1975). Identifying the factors that modify learning in acutely traumatized groups will provide much needed evidence about both risk and protective factors. To date, no further data have emerged in human populations that help us better characterize the nature of the acute stress response and how this might be a risk factor for PTSD. Obviously, a variety of neurobiological systems would be of interest.

PTSD as a Transitional Disorder

The preliminary data discussed in the previous section highlight the need for better characterization of the nature of the acute stress response and its transition into the range of psychiatric disorders that emerge after traumatic exposure. The critical factor may turn out to be not the traumatic event itself, but rather the individual's ability to modulate his or her acute stress response and to restore psychological and biological homeostasis. Thus, PTSD may be a disorder of transition rather than a specific stress disorder. In other words, the critical issue is not that individuals with PTSD have a greater acute stress response; rather, it is that they are unable to modulate this reaction.

The impact of family psychiatric history, prior psychiatric disorder, and peritraumatic dissociation on this transitional process is of particular importance to the further understanding of the neurobiology of PTSD. Also, the very preliminary finding that subjects who went on to develop PTSD had a lower cortisol rise (McFarlane et al. 1997; Resnick et al. 1995) emphasizes the need for much greater understanding of the nature of the traumatic stress response that leads to PTSD. The interest in hypocortisolemia as a possible factor leading to decreased hippocampal volume in patients with PTSD highlights the necessity for more careful systematic research around this question (McEwen and Magarinos 1997; Sopolsky 1996; Yehuda 1997). Furthermore, the data presented in this chapter emphasize the importance of looking at the progression and changes in PTSD over time and the interplay of risk factors and protective counterparts.

The conceptual issue of the nature of the relationship between acute distress and PTSD begs the question as to where many of the risk factors in PTSD exert their effect. In other words, PTSD may involve a failure of the resolution of the acute stress response or, in the more toxic forms of posttraumatic adaptation, a progressive recruitment of instabilities of the underlying neurobiological systems. This possibility raises many interesting questions about the relationships among the acute psychological state of an individual, his or her neurobiological systems, and the capacity for preventive treatment interventions to be of benefit in the period immediately after a traumatic experience. The ability of an individual to modulate their distress at these times may be critical in determining the long-term outcome. It may be that during this phase there is a secondary series of modifications of underlying memory structures that further increases the risk of chronic poor outcomes.

Investigation of this transitional stage may also be of particular

importance in understanding why some individuals who experience traumatic events develop PTSD over time, whereas others develop conditions such as major depression and panic. The nature of
the acute stress response and progressive modifications of the individual's affective state during this transitional stage may be other
risk factors that lead to these different patterns of adaptation. It is
possible that during this phase there are general and specific risk
factors for psychiatric disorders and other specific conditions. In
other words, there may be a general vulnerability to dysregulation,
whose pattern is then determined by specific underlying vulnerability markers or risk factors that can be defined at the time of the
traumatic experience.

This review of the risk factors operating at the time of the trauma
that influence the nature of the acute stress response shows that,
from both the conceptual and investigational points of view, this
field is in its infancy. This begs the question as to the models that
may be of some use in better characterizing these risk factors.

Several Models for Future Investigation

Kindling

Post and colleagues (1997) have highlighted how behavioral sensitization and kindling models of memory functioning explain increased behavioral outputs and the progressive evolution in the
biochemical and neuroanatomic substrates involved in PTSD.
These authors emphasized in particular the importance of amygdala kindling in this process. The process of kindling is a complex
spatiotemporal cascade of neurobiological events involving
changes in gene expression. Post et al. hypothesize that there are
two dimensions to this process. The first involves the model of kin-
dled seizures that increase in severity and spontaneity. The second
involves a secondary compensatory and potentially adaptive
mechanism of quenching this hyperexcitability.

The work on kindling provides a very useful model for systematic investigation. It serves as a method of examining the differential inputs of different risk factors at this acute stage and the nature

of their contribution (some may have aggravating effects, whereas others may have protective effects).

Stress-Induced Oscillation

A second conceptual model for the disruption of this transitional phase in PTSD is stress-induced oscillation. Antelman and colleagues (1997) have highlighted the usefulness of this process in understanding the instabilities within neurobiological systems that may explain aspects of the onset of PTSD. This group's research has demonstrated that repeated, intermittent exposure to either pharmacological or nondrug stresses can induce both neurochemical and behavioral oscillation or cycling that is an alternative pattern of decreases and increases in the response to subsequent treatment or stress.

Such oscillation occurs in biological systems that have reached or are approaching their physiological limits. It represents a process of dynamic homeostasis of systems that are approaching overload. This phenomenon has been demonstrated in a variety of neurobiological systems, including the dopaminergic, serotonergic, and hypothalamic CRF (corticotropin-releasing factor) systems. Given the severity of the impact of acute traumatic stresses and the probability that most of these systems are functioning close to their biological limits, it can be inferred that this model has relevance to an understanding of PTSD. Thus, risk factors might be the demonstrable characteristics that influence the range and capacity of response of such neurobiological systems.

Supporting Phenomenological Evidence

The importance of kindling, quenching, and stress-induced oscillation to the transitional shifts in an individual's acute stress response derives from a variety of work on the determinants of the course of PTSD. A wide range of studies have demonstrated that the severity of current PTSD symptoms is related in large part to the more recent nontraumatic life events to which individuals have been exposed (Koopman et al. 1994; McFarlane 1989; Yehuda et al. 1995). The implication is that such secondary life events can play

a major role in influencing the dynamic state of an individual's biological system and that, therefore, the nature of the posttraumatic
environment is an important secondary risk factor.

In addition, the impact of the distress caused by the illness itself
should not be underestimated as a secondary risk factor. Hence,
sources of endogenous distress might be important contributors to
the destabilization of biological systems as secondary life events.
Some patients comment that flashbacks can be more distressing
than the primary traumatic experience. As with affective disorders,
this implies that rapid and early control of symptoms may have
major implications for the prognosis for PTSD. Thus, treatment-seeking behavior may be an important secondary risk factor.
However, Kessler and colleagues (1995) suggest that if the PTSD
has not resolved within 72 months, there is a very substantial probability that the disorder will be chronic. Sixty percent of individuals will experience a remission, and in most of these cases the
remission will occur in the first year. These data highlight that
there may be time windows when these modulating factors might
operate and that these factors may have their greatest effect in close
proximity to the trauma.

Pynoos and colleagues (1997), in an interesting animal model of
PTSD, found that repeated reexposure to traumatic reminders was
a powerful predictor of the emergence of the behavior suggestive
of PTSD. In contrast, the acute stressor, when presented in isola-
tion, appeared to prime the animal. Clinicians recognize how exposure to triggers can cause major exacerbations in individuals'
symptoms. It is possible to see how traumatic reminders may have
a progressively destabilizing effect in the early stages of the disorder and adverse consequences for the prognosis. Thus, important
secondary risk factors modifying the acute stress response are the
degree of the individual distress, the prevalence of triggers, and
the nature of posttraumatic adversity.

Conclusion

One of the challenges in conceptualizing the role of risk factors operating around the time of traumatic events is to understand the

complex interactions among these risk factors and how they modulate the normal process of adaptation to such experiences. As the nature of traumatic memories becomes better understood—in particular the neurobiological substrates involving declarative and nondeclarative memory—it may be possible to further our understanding of the variability of these processes. However, it is important not to assume that there is a direct correspondence between these normal processes of adaptation and the nature of the abnormalities in PTSD. These normal processes form the templates on which various models of destabilization can be superimposed. The emerging research highlights the importance of time as a critical dimension in the emergence of posttraumatic syndromes.

Prospective studies are critical to describe the exact points at which various risk factors may operate in PTSD. The range of findings about the role of dissociation in this disorder highlights how retrospective recall may lead to oversimplification of the way that acute risk factors operate. Further investigation of these processes has major implications for treatment of individuals with this condition in its early stages and the possibilities of primary prevention. The exact timing to achieve the optimal benefit needs to be determined.

Posttraumatic stress disorder has a significant rate of natural remission in a number of cases. This emphasizes the importance of understanding the factors that might influence the timing of the remission and the extent to which a template is laid down in close proximity to the stressor. Similarly, the factors that might exacerbate the symptoms or modify them in the course of the disorder need to be investigated separately.

References

American Psychiatric Association: Diagnostic and Statistical Manual of Mental Disorders, 3rd Edition. Washington, DC, American Psychiatric Press, 1980

American Psychiatric Association: Diagnostic and Statistical Manual of Mental Disorders, 4th Edition. Washington, DC, American Psychiatric Press, 1994

Antelman SM, Caggiula A, Gershon S, et al: Stressor-induced oscillation: a possible model of the bidirectional symptoms in PTSD. Ann N Y Acad Sci 821:296–304, 1997

Atchison M, McFarlane AC: A review of dissociation and dissociative disorders. Aust N Z J Psychiatry 28:591–599, 1994

Barton KA, Blanchard EB, Hickling EJ: Antecedents and consequences of acute stress disorder among motor vehicle accident victims. Behav Res Ther 34:805–813, 1996

Bremner JD, Krystal JH, Southwick SM, et al: Functional neuroanatomical correlates of the effects of stress on memory. J Trauma Stress 8:527–553, 1995

Breslau N, Davis GC, Anderski P, et al: Traumatic events and posttraumatic stress disorder in an urban population of young adults. Arch Gen Psychiatry 48:216–222, 1991

Breuer J, Freud S: Studies on hysteria (1893–1895), in The Standard Edition of the Complete Psychological Works of Sigmund Freud, Vol 2. Translated and edited by Strachey J. London, Hogarth Press, 1955, pp 1–319

Cahill L: The neurobiology of emotionally influenced memory: implications for understanding traumatic memory. Ann N Y Acad Sci 821:238–246, 1997

Cahill L, Babinsky R, Markowitsch HJ, et al: The amygdala and emotional memory. Nature 377(6547):295–296, 1995

DeFazio VJ, Rustin SX, Diamond A: Symptom development in Vietnam era veterans. Am J Orthopsychiatry 45:158–163, 1975

Figley CR: Psychosocial adjustment among Vietnam veterans: an overview of the research, in Stress Disorders Among Vietnam Veterans. Edited by Figley CR. New York, Brunner/Mazel, 1978, pp 57–70

Foa EB: Psychological processes related to recovery from a trauma and an effective treatment for PTSD. Ann N Y Acad Sci 821:410–424, 1997

Gold PE, McGaugh JL: In Short-Term Memory. Edited by Deutsch D, Deutsch JA. New York, Academic Press, 1975, pp 355–378

Grinker RR, Spiegel JP: Men Under Stress. Philadelphia, PA, Blakiston, 1945

Haan N: A tripartite model of ego functioning: value and clinical research application. J Nerv Ment Dis 148:14–30, 1969

Holen A: A Long-Term Outcome Study of Survivors From Disaster. Oslo, Norway, University of Oslo Press, 1990

Janet P: Problems Psychologiques de L'Emotion. Review Neurology 17: 1551–1687, 1909

Janet P: Psychological Healing, Vols 1 and 2. New York, Macmillan, 1925

Kessler RC, Sonnega A, Bromet E, et al: Posttraumatic stress disorder in the National Comorbidity Survey. Arch Gen Psychiatry 52:1048–1060, 1995

Koopman C, Classen C, Spiegel D: Predictors of posttraumatic stress symptoms among survivors of the Oakland/Berkeley, Calif., firestorm. Am J Psychiatry 151:888–894, 1994

Lazarus RS, Folkman S: Stress, Appraisal and Coping. New York, Springer, 1984

Leed E: No Man's Land. London, Cambridge University Press, 1979

Lundin T: Psychological morbidity after the Estonia Ferry Disaster. Paper presented at the 2nd World Conference of the International Society for Traumatic Stress Studies, Jerusalem, June 1996

Malt UF, Olafsen OM: Psychological appraisal and emotional response to physical injury: a clinical, phenomenological study of 109 adults. Psychiatry in Medicine 10:117–134, 1992

Malt UF, Blikra G, Hoivik B: The three-year biopsychosocial outcome of 551 hospitalized accidentally injured adults. Acta Psychiatr Scand 80:84–93, 1989

Marmar CR, Weiss DS, Schlenger WE, et al: Peritraumatic dissociation and posttraumatic stress in male Vietnam theater veterans. Am J Psychiatry 151:902–907, 1994

Mayou R, Bryant B, Duthie R: Psychiatric consequences of road traffic accidents. BMJ 307:647–651, 1993

McEwen B, Magarinos AM: Stress effects on morphology and function of the hippocampus. Ann N Y Acad Sci 821:271–284, 1997

McFarlane AC: The aetiology of post-traumatic morbidity: predisposing, precipitating and perpetuating factors. Br J Psychiatry 154:221–228, 1989

McFarlane AC: Avoidance and intrusion in posttraumatic stress disorder. J Nerv Ment Dis 180:439–445, 1992

McFarlane AC: The prevalence and longitudinal course of PTSD: implications for the neurobiological models of PTSD. Ann N Y Acad Sci 821: 10–23, 1997

McFarlane AC, de Girolamo G: The nature of traumatic stressors and the epidemiology of posttraumatic reactions, in Traumatic Stress: The Effects of Overwhelming Experience on Mind, Body and Society. Edited by van der Kolk BA, McFarlane AC, Weisaeth L. New York, Guilford, 1996, pp 129–154

McFarlane AC, Atchison M, Yehuda R: The acute stress response following motor vehicle accidents and its relation to PTSD. Ann N Y Acad Sci 821:437–441, 1997

Norris FH: Epidemiology of trauma: frequency and impact of different potentially traumatic events on different demographic groups. J Consult Clin Psychol 60:409–418, 1992

Pearlin LI, Schooler C: The structure of coping. J Health Soc Behav 22: 337–356, 1978

Post RM, Weiss SRB, Smith M, et al: Kindling vs quenching: implications for the treatment of PTSD. Ann N Y Acad Sci 821:285–295, 1997

Pynoos RS, Steinberg AM, Ornitz EM, et al: Issues in the developmental neurobiology of traumatic stress. Ann N Y Acad Sci 821:176–193, 1997

Rachman S: Fear and Courage. New York, WH Freeman, 1990

Raphael B, Wilson J, Meldrum L, et al: Acute preventative interventions, in Traumatic Stress: The Effects of Overwhelming Experience on Mind, Body and Society. Edited by van der Kolk BA, McFarlane AC, Weisaeth L. New York, Guilford, 1996, pp 463–479

Resnick HS, Yehuda R, Pitman RK, et al: Effect of previous trauma on acute plasma cortisol level following rape. Am J Psychiatry 152: 1675–1677, 1995

Saigh P: Pre- and postinvasion anxiety in Lebanon. Behavior Therapy 15: 185–190, 1984

Shalev AY: Posttraumatic stress disorder among injured survivors of terrorist attack: predictive value of early intrusion and avoidance symptoms. J Nerv Ment Dis 180:505–509, 1992

Shalev A: Treatment failure in acute PTSD: lessons learned about the complexity of the disorder. Ann N Y Acad Sci 821:372–387, 1997

Shalev A, Munitz H: Combat stress reaction, in Manual of Disaster Medicine. Edited by Ries ND, Dolev E. Berlin, Springer-Verlag, 1989, pp 169–182

Shalev AY, Peri T, Canetti L, et al: Predictors of PTSD in injured trauma survivors: a prospective study. Am J Psychiatry 153:219–225, 1996

Solomon Z: Somatic complaints, stress reaction and post-traumatic stress disorder: a 3-year follow-up study. Behav Med 14:179–186, 1988

Solomon Z: Characteristic psychiatric symptomatology in PTSD veterans: a three year follow-up. Psychol Med 19:927–936, 1989

Solomon Z: Combat Stress Reaction: The Enduring Toll of War. New York, Plenum, 1993

Solomon Z: The Psychological Aftermath of Combat Stress Reaction: An 18-Year Follow-up. Technical Report. Jerusalem, Israeli Ministry of Defense, 1994

Solomon Z, Kleinhauz M: War induced psychic trauma: an 18-year follow-up of Israeli veterans. Am J Orthopsychiatry 66:152–160, 1996

Solomon Z, Mikulincer M: Combat stress reaction, posttraumatic stress disorder and somatic complaints among Israeli soldiers. J Psychosom Res 31:131–137, 1987

Solomon Z, Mikulincer M, Kotler M: A two year follow-up of somatic complaints among Israeli combat stress reaction casualties. J Psychosom Res 31:463–469, 1987

Solomon Z, Avitzur E, Mikulincer M: Coping styles and post-war psychopathology among Israeli soldiers. Personality and Individual Differences 11:451–456, 1990a

Solomon Z, Mikulincer M, Habershaim N: Life-events, coping strategies, social resources, and somatic complaints among combat stress reaction casualties. Br J Med Psychol 63:137–148, 1990b

Solomon Z, Laor N, McFarlane AC: Acute posttraumatic reactions in soldiers and civilians, in Traumatic Stress: The Effects of Overwhelming Experience on Mind, Body and Society. Edited by van der Kolk BA, McFarlane AC, Weisaeth L. New York, Guilford, 1996, pp 102–114

Sopolsky RM: Why stress is bad for the brain (comment). Science 273:749, 1996

Southwick SM, Bremner D, Krystal JH, et al: Psychobiologic research in posttraumatic stress disorder. Psychiatr Clin North Am 17:251–264, 1994

Spiegel D: Dissociation and trauma, in American Psychiatric Press Review of Psychiatry: Vol 10. Edited by Tasman A, Goldfinger SM. Washington, DC, American Psychiatric Press, 1991, pp 261–275

Spiegel D: Trauma, dissociation and memory. Ann N Y Acad Sci 821: 225–237, 1997

Spurrell MT, McFarlane AC: Life-events and psychiatric symptoms in a general psychiatry clinic—the role of intrusion and avoidance. Br J Med Psychol 68:333–340, 1995

Tromp S, Koss MP, Figueredo AJ, et al: Are rape memories different? A comparison of rape, other unpleasant and pleasant memories among employed women. J Trauma Stress 8:607–627, 1995

van der Kolk BA, Fisler R: Dissociation and the perceptual nature of traumatic memories: review and experimental confirmation. J Trauma Stress 8:505–525, 1995

van der Kolk BA, Weisaeth L, van der Hart O: History of trauma in psychiatry, in Traumatic Stress: The Effects of Overwhelming Experience on Mind, Body and Society. Edited by van der Kolk BA, McFarlane AC, Weisaeth L. New York, Guilford, 1996, pp 47–74

Weisaeth L: The stressors and the post-traumatic stress syndrome after an industrial disaster. Acta Psychiatr Scand Suppl 355:25–37, 1989a

Weisaeth L: A study of behavioural responses to an industrial disaster. Acta Psychiatr Scand Suppl 355:13–24, 1989b

Weisaeth L: PTSD: vulnerability and protective factors. Baillieres Clinical Psychiatry 2:217–228, 1996

Weiss DS, Marmar CR, Metzler TJ, et al: Predicting symptomatic distress in emergency services personnel. J Consult Clin Psychol 63:361–368, 1995

World Health Organization: ICD Classification of Mental and Behavioural Disorders: Clinical Descriptions and Diagnostic Guidelines. Geneva, World Health Organization, 1992

Yehuda R: Stress and glucocorticoid (letter). Science 275:1662, 1997

Yehuda R, Antelman SM: Criteria for rationally evaluating animal models of post-traumatic stress disorder. Biol Psychiatry 33:479–486, 1993

Yehuda R, McFarlane AC: Conflict between current knowledge about PTSD and its original conceptual basis. Am J Psychiatry 152:1705–1713, 1995

Yehuda R, Boisoneau D, Lowy MT, et al: Dose-response changes in plasma cortisol and lymphocyte glucocorticoid receptors following dexamethasone administration in combat veterans with and without posttraumatic stress disorder. Arch Gen Psychiatry 52:583–593, 1995

Chapter 9

Personality as a Risk Factor for PTSD

Paula P. Schnurr, Ph.D., and Melanie J. Vielhauer, Ph.D.

The stimulus for this chapter, as well as the book in which it appears, is that many people are likely to experience a traumatic event but few develop posttraumatic stress disorder (PTSD). According to a large national study, only 8% of traumatized men and 20% of traumatized women developed PTSD at some point after traumatic exposure (Kessler et al. 1995). Since the introduction of PTSD into the diagnostic nomenclature (American Psychiatric Association 1980), the field of traumatic stress studies has undergone a significant conceptual shift in how to interpret the low prevalence of PTSD given the high prevalence of trauma—from relatively strong deemphasis of the role of antecedent factors (e.g., Foy et al. 1984) to increasing recognition that the likelihood of PTSD varies as a function of characteristics of an individual prior to trauma (e.g., Breslau et al. 1991; Green et al. 1990). In fact, even the idea that PTSD is a *normative,* as opposed to abnormal, response to a traumatic stressor has been questioned (Yehuda and McFarlane 1995).

In this chapter, we review evidence relevant to the hypothesis that antecedent personality characteristics function as risk and protective factors in the development of PTSD or posttraumatic symptoms. The review is comprehensive but selective and favors

Preparation of this manuscript was supported by a Department of Veterans Affairs Merit Review grant to the first author. We would like to thank Alison Paris for bibliographic and administrative assistance and Dr. Matthew Friedman for helpful comments.

empirical over case study material. We begin by discussing methodological issues that affect the interpretation of risk factors as causes. We next provide a theoretical framework for understanding personality and how it could function as a risk factor. We then review the literature on the association between personality and PTSD.

Our focus is on normal personality and personality disorder and not factors that might influence personality development (e.g., childhood emotional abuse). We do not address individual differences in general, such as those involving gender and education, despite the fact that these and many other characteristics are associated with increased or decreased risk of PTSD (e.g., Breslau et al. 1991; Green et al. 1990; Kessler et al. 1995; Kulka et al. 1990). Because of space considerations, we have excluded references to works on posttraumatic reactions other than PTSD; this means that we do not discuss some fascinating and insightful historical material by authors such as Brill and Beebe (1955). However, we encourage readers to consult older sources for clinically rich information.

Methodological Considerations

Risk factors are variables that are associated with the occurrence of a disease outcome. Sometimes the term *protective factor* is used to indicate a variable that is associated with relatively lower disease occurrence; here we use *risk factor* to apply both to variables that have risk-increasing effects and to those that have risk-decreasing effects. The term describes causes for an outcome as well as markers for causes, which are also known as *risk indicators* (Ahlbom and Norell 1990). The interpretation of a risk factor as a cause is difficult—especially if experimental control over a presumed cause is not possible, as in the case of traumatic exposure and PTSD. Virtually all of the literature on personality and PTSD comes from cross-sectional, correlational investigations in which personality and PTSD are measured simultaneously.

For example, Breslau and colleagues (1991) assessed a group of young adults for both personality and PTSD and found that neuroticism was positively associated with lifetime PTSD. How are we to understand this association? One possible interpretation assigns a causal role to the personality factor: neuroticism may predispose traumatized individuals to develop PTSD. But in making this interpretation we must consider the issues involved in making a causal inference from nonexperimental data, an approach that represents a general problem in understanding the etiology of PTSD and other psychiatric disorders. We discuss these issues only briefly because they are likely to be familiar to most readers (see Cook and Campbell 1979 for an expanded discussion).

One issue is what is known as the "third variable" problem. Neuroticism may not influence reactions to trauma but may be associated with PTSD because some factors that influence likelihood of PTSD also influence personality development. A possible candidate is a prior trauma history, which is associated with increased likelihood of war zone–related PTSD (D. W. King et al. 1996). Note that we mention trauma history only for illustration and are not proposing that a prior trauma history causes increased neuroticism. Also note that in this case personality would be a risk indicator of PTSD.

Another issue is that temporal order may be difficult to infer from cross-sectional data, so that what appears to be a cause actually may be an outcome. Neuroticism may be associated with PTSD because having PTSD may make people more neurotic, or at least more likely to endorse items on a neuroticism scale. The problem may be especially likely in studies of chronic PTSD because having an Axis I disorder may have profound long-term effects (Friedman and Rosenheck 1996).

A related issue is that cross-sectional data are uninformative regarding longitudinal patterns of relationships among causes and effects. Personality may be both a cause and an effect of PTSD: neuroticism may predispose traumatized individuals to develop PTSD, chronic PTSD in turn may increase neuroticism, and this transactional relationship may recur over time. A cross-sectional snapshot of trauma survivors will fail to reveal the complex interplay.

In the absence of experimental control and random assignment, these interpretive difficulties may be attenuated by the use of statistical and methodological procedures. Multivariate data analytic strategies increase control over potential third variables. The use of pretraumatic personality measures helps rule out problems of temporal order, and longitudinal designs permit inferences about transactional relationships. Nonetheless, interpretive difficulties may remain. All relevant variables may not have been measured and included in a study that uses multivariate statistical control. Also, third variables need to be considered, even in a study that uses pretraumatic personality measures (e.g., Card 1983; Schnurr et al. 1993). The ideal nonexperimental design incorporates multivariate statistical procedures, pretraumatic personality measures, and multiple posttraumatic assessments. We are unaware of any study that incorporates all of these features. Instead, most findings from studies of the relationship between personality and PTSD are open to multiple interpretations. We thus encourage readers to exercise caution in reading not just our review but also the articles on which it is based.

All of the foregoing methodological concerns arise from the fact that the entire body of literature on personality and PTSD is based on correlational data. An additional issue that should be kept in mind when reading this literature is the nature of the outcome that is being predicted. In general, a study that focuses on lifetime PTSD as an outcome provides information about the development of PTSD, whereas a study that focuses on current PTSD provides information about the maintenance of PTSD, especially if the study population has chronic PTSD. Both types of studies are useful, but they should be distinguished from each other. An exemplary approach to making this distinction comes from a set of studies by Breslau, who first examined risk factors for lifetime PTSD (Breslau et al. 1991) and then examined risk factors for chronicity among individuals who had lifetime PTSD (Breslau and Davis 1992). One drawback of this approach is the reduced statistical power for examining risk factors for chronicity; a variable that is actually predictive of both the development and the maintenance of PTSD may appear to be a risk factor for lifetime PTSD but not chronic PTSD because the sample size for the latter analysis will, of necessity, be smaller. Nevertheless, it is unfortunate that, as far as we know, no other studies of risk factors for PTSD have followed a similar strategy. Thus, there is little clarity regarding the question of whether risk factors relevant to the development of PTSD differ from those relevant to the maintenance of the disorder.

What Is Personality?

Laypersons and professionals alike view personality as a constellation of attributes, or traits, that describe, explain, and predict an individual's behavior. Despite numerous differences among theorists about the particular organization and function of personality (see Lindzey et al. 1988), most agree that the trait concept implies consistency of behavior. In recent years, much of the research on personality has centered on determining the structure and organization of personality. The general consensus seems to be that personality structure can be described by a relatively small number of broad trait dimensions. The predominant number of dimensions is thought by many to be five—neuroticism, extraversion, intellect/openness to experience, conscientiousness, and agreeableness (Goldberg 1990; McCrae and Costa 1996).

Another topic in personality research is the question of continuity between normal personality and personality disorder. The implication of DSM-IV (American Psychiatric Association 1994) is that personality disorder is categorically distinct from normal personality, although evidence tends to support the utility of conceptualizing both normal and disordered personality as points along continua that represent lesser and greater amounts of basic trait dimensions. Watson and colleagues (1994) provide an excellent summary of the research on personality structure and how the structure relates to the study of psychopathology. They offer their own structural model, relating it to models of normal personality, and emphasize how many traits are relevant to Axis I and II disorders, (e.g., neuroticism consists of traits that include anxiety, depression, guilt, emotional lability, and somatic complaints). (For extended discussion, see the special issue of the *Journal of Abnormal Psychology* edited by Watson and Clark [1994].)

We mention these issues in basic personality research only to provide readers with a sense of the broader context in which relevant knowledge about personality and PTSD exists. Adequate discussion of these and other questions about the *structure* of personality is beyond the scope of this chapter and, we believe, unnecessary for understanding the relationship between personality and reactions to traumatic events. What is necessary, however, is familiarity with a model of *process*: how personality traits relate to behavior, which we define in terms of both observable actions and unobservable thoughts and feelings. Any discussion of the literature on personality as a risk factor for PTSD must be grounded in a reasonable explanation of how personality could increase or decrease the likelihood of PTSD following trauma.

As noted above, traditional conceptualizations have viewed personality as an organized set of traits that are consistently expressed in behavior across situations and over time. It is assumed that a high level of a trait leads to frequent behaviors reflecting that trait (e.g., a high level of shyness leads to extreme discomfort in and avoidance of social situations) and minimal participation in those situations that cannot be avoided. In fact, the correspondence between traits and behavior is far from perfect. There is, however, good consistency in intraindividual patterns of response to different situations, or "if . . . then . . . situation-behavior profiles" (Mischel and Shoda 1995). For example, a shy child who becomes irritable and hostile in social situations with peers but withdrawn and docile in social situations with adults is likely to display this pattern on repeated occasions.

Mischel and Shoda's (1995) theory of a "Cognitive-Affective Personality System" serves to explain the processes underlying individual differences in cognitive, affective, and behavioral reactions to situations. According to the theory, individual differences in behavior result from the interaction of five types of person variables, which they label "cognitive-affective units":

- *Encodings,* or categories for representing the self, people, events, and situations
- *Expectancies and beliefs*

- *Affects,* which encompass feelings, emotions, affective re-sponses, and physiological reactions
- *Goals and values*
- *Competencies and self-regulatory plans*

Individuals may differ in both the cognitive-affective units them-selves and the way in which these units are organized and relate to psychological features of situations. In particular, persons may dif-fer predictably in if . . . then . . . situation-behavior profiles—that is, in the patterns of activation that occur in response to configura-tions of situational features across situations. Both the cogni-tive-affective units and their organization and activation are influenced by temperamental/genetic and situational influences. Mischel and Shoda provide support for their model by presenting the results of a computer-generated simulation that reproduced two of the major findings of personality research: variability in mean trait levels and stability of situation-behavior profiles.

Within a theory that is so fundamentally based on the distinct-ness of individuals, dispositions are a "characteristic cognitive af-fective processing structure that underlies, and generates, distinctive processing dynamics" (Mischel and Shoda 1995, p. 257). The structure refers to a characteristic set of units and their organi-zation; the dynamics are the patterns of activation that are gener-ated in response to particular situations. Individuals who have similar processing structures and processing dynamics have a sim-ilar processing disposition—what we would call a personality type. Yet the theory is not reductionistic. On the contrary, Mischel and Shoda emphasize the importance of understanding meaning: "The ultimate goal becomes to articulate the psychological struc-ture that underlies this organization within the personality sys-tem" (p. 259).

One desirable property of the Cognitive-Affective Personality System is that the network formulation on which it is based is con-sistent with current theories of information processing, known as "connectionist" or "neural network" models (Davis 1992). Al-though this system is not explicitly proposed as a neural network model, such a formulation could be added, for example, to model the development of activation patterns among cognitive-affective units. The network-based formulation also is consistent with Foa and colleagues' (1989) information processing model of PTSD, which is based on the concept of fear networks that contain fear-relevant stimulus and response information in memory. A fear structure could be understood within the Cognitive-Affective Personality System as a particular configuration of cognitive-affective units that is activated in response to situational features that have come to indicate danger to an individual.

Using the theoretical framework provided by Mischel and Shoda (1995), we offer the following example to illustrate how personality could affect reactions to trauma. Consider the hypothetical case of two women, each of whom is raped by a single, unknown perpetrator who breaks into her locked home and threatens her with a weapon. Each women encodes the situation as a threat to physical integrity in which she is powerless and experiences extreme fear as a result. However, because of temperamental and prior developmental experiences, the women differ in terms of the processing structure and processing dynamics of their individual personality systems. For one woman, situations that engender powerlessness and fear trigger anger and the expectation that no one will help her, so she avoids talking to others about the rape and buys a gun to protect herself in the future. For the other woman, situations that engender powerlessness and fear trigger the need to seek comfort from others and the expectation that others can help, so she reaches out to friends, goes to therapy, and joins a rape support group. We might expect that the first woman would be more likely than the second to develop PTSD. We also might expect the first woman to score low on a personality scale that measures need for affiliation, but this would not necessarily be true. In general, both women could have the same affiliative needs, but those needs could be differentially aroused in response to situational features.

This latter point has important implications for the study of how pretraumatic personality relates to posttraumatic outcomes. It suggests that simply measuring an overall amount of a trait in relation to PTSD—the strategy used in all of the studies we review—could lead to Type II errors in making inferences about that trait's potential as a risk factor. Keeping this point in mind, we now turn to the empirical literature on the association between personality and PTSD. We review first cross-sectional studies and then the few prospective studies completed to date. None of this literature lends itself to discussion in terms of cognitive-affective units. However, we return to Mischel and Shoda's (1995) model in our concluding comments in an attempt to suggest a basis for such integration in future research.

Review of the Evidence

Cross-Sectional Studies

Personality Profiles and PTSD

One line of investigation in the study of personality and PTSD is based on assessments of personality profiles with instruments such as the Minnesota Multiphasic Personality Inventory (MMPI; Hathaway and McKinley 1967) and the Millon Clinical Multiaxial Inventory (MCMI; Millon 1987). Profile studies represent a sizable literature on the relationship between personality and PTSD. Although the MMPI in particular is typically used as a diagnostic indicator of PTSD (e.g., Keane et al. 1984) and not as a way to assess risk for PTSD, we include cross-sectional MMPI and MCMI studies in our review and encourage readers to use caution in making causal judgments.

Studies of combat veterans and survivors of civilian trauma have generally shown that individuals with PTSD, relative to both well-adjusted and psychiatric control subjects, have MMPI profile elevations in the clinical range (i.e., T scores greater than 70; e.g., Engdahl et al. 1991; Keane et al. 1984; Koretzky and Peck 1990; Orr et al. 1990; but see also Silver and Salamone-Genovese 1991). With regard to MMPI profile shape, results of many studies have suggested that a 2-8-[7]/8-2-[7] configuration with an elevated F-scale score is characteristic of Vietnam combat veterans diagnosed with PTSD (e.g., Foy et al. 1984; Keane et al. 1984; Orr et al. 1990; but see also Silver and Salamone-Genovese 1991). Similarly, investigators have often found a 2-8/8-2 modal code type for individuals with PTSD in clinical samples of both adult and child civilian trauma victims (e.g., Frederick 1985; Koretzky and Peck 1990). The 2-8/8-2 profile is associated with characteristics such as social introversion, interpersonal hypersensitivity, lack of meaningful social involvements, dependence, lack of assertiveness, irritability, resentfulness, and suspiciousness (Butcher and Williams 1992). Individuals with this code type are likely to fear losing control of their emotions and to deny undesirable emotions. They are unlikely to express themselves in a direct manner but may exhibit negative emotions during dissociative episodes. These characteristics are distinguished from the more acute symptoms that are also associated with this particular profile configuration (e.g., agitation, jumpiness, sleep disturbance, inability to concentrate).

Similar to MMPI findings, results from studies that have used the MCMI demonstrate that individuals with PTSD typically have elevated profiles, relative to those of individuals without PTSD (e.g., Robert et al. 1985). With striking consistency, the profile most commonly associated with PTSD has been the passive-aggressive/avoidant code type (2-8/8-2), with elevations in the clinically significant range (e.g., Hyer et al. 1990, 1994b; Robert et al. 1985).

The likelihood that the 2-8/8-2 MMPI/MCMI profile is a risk factor for PTSD is attenuated by findings that this profile accounts for a relatively small proportion of the code types in PTSD samples (e.g., Gaston et al. 1996). Also, the 2-8/8-2 type does not adequately characterize PTSD-positive veterans from earlier eras, such as World War II and Korean conflict former prisoners of war (POWs). Findings have consistently revealed a 1-2-[3]/2-1-[3] mean profile for this population (e.g., Engdahl et al. 1991; Sutker et al. 1991), suggestive of passive-dependence, hostility, irritability, self-consciousness, introversion, somatization, and repression (Butcher and Williams 1992). Furthermore, the 2-8/8-2 profile is not unique to PTSD, and the profile configurations of individuals with PTSD and psychiatric control subjects are often similar in shape, despite the relative elevations associated with PTSD (e.g., Foy et al. 1984; Keane et al. 1984).

A greater impediment to viewing the 2-8/8-2 profile or any other profile as a risk factor for PTSD is evidence suggesting that the profile elevations in PTSD reflect a change subsequent to the development of chronic PTSD. Combat veterans with current PTSD have higher mean profiles than combatants who have recovered from PTSD, although both groups have elevated profiles relative to former combatants with other psychiatric diagnoses or with no psychiatric disorders (Engdahl et al. 1991). Gaston and colleagues (1996) found that treatment-seeking civilians with chronic PTSD (i.e., duration of at least 6 months) had significantly higher MMPI profiles than did either treatment-seeking civilians with acute PTSD or non–treatment-seeking control subjects with panic disorder. The acute PTSD and panic groups did not differ, and the observed elevations in the acute group were just above the normal range (i.e., approximately 70). Also, 14% of the chronic PTSD group had a 2-8/8-2 profile, compared with 5% of the acute PTSD group (a difference for which we compute the probability to be $P < 0.05$).

Overall, data from the cross-sectional investigations that have used the MMPI and MCMI do not lend support to the possibility that personality is a risk factor for PTSD. All cross-sectional investigations make it difficult to infer etiological relationships, but the MMPI data actually suggest that personality changes result from the development of PTSD, at least in its chronic form.

Personality Disorder and PTSD

In this subsection, we review empirical studies on the association between PTSD and Axis II disorders. Selected studies examining PTSD and broadly defined childhood behavioral difficulties are included because of the role of such difficulties in the diagnosis of antisocial personality disorder and their relevance to the question of whether pretraumatic personality is associated with risk of PTSD.

Most studies that have examined the association between PTSD and personality disorder have targeted antisocial personality disorder. Studies that included other Axis II disorders in an assessment battery are inconclusive. Kluznik and colleagues (1986) found no relationship between PTSD and antisocial or "labile" disorders in World War II former POWs. Blanchard and colleagues (1995) found no relationship between PTSD and antisocial, borderline, obsessive-compulsive, paranoid, avoidant, or dependent disorders, nor between PTSD and a summary measure of any personality disorder, in motor vehicle accident survivors. Wilson and Krauss (1985) found a few correlations between subscales of an inventory that measured PTSD and associated features and scales that measured antisocial, paranoid, and narcissistic behaviors, but only narcissism was correlated with all PTSD subscales.

In contrast, large epidemiological studies have documented an association between PTSD and antisocial personality disorder in both civilian (Helzer et al. 1987; Kessler et al. 1995) and veteran (Barrett et al. 1996; Kulka et al. 1990) samples. Also, Resnick and colleagues (1989) found an association between PTSD and adult antisocial behaviors in veterans. Only a few, much smaller, studies with less-representative samples have failed to find an association between PTSD and antisocial personality disorder (Blanchard et al. 1995; Green et al. 1990; Kluznik et al. 1986). It is interesting, however, that two of the studies that failed to find an association attempted to diagnose pretraumatic antisocial personality, albeit retrospectively (Blanchard et al. 1995; Green et al. 1990). This raises the question of whether the observed associations between PTSD and antisocial personality disorder are the result of PTSD's increasing the risk of subsequently developing antisocial personality disorder. Attempting to answer the question actually raises several others because of complex relationships among childhood behavior problems, trauma, and adult antisocial behavior.

Retrospectively assessed childhood behavior problems have been linked to both PTSD (Barrett et al. 1996; Helzer et al. 1987; Kulka et al. 1990) and traumatic exposure (Barrett et al. 1996); only Resnick and colleagues (1989) failed to find either association. Sorting out the potential interrelationships among these variables is best accomplished by structural equation modeling, which D. W.

King and colleagues (1996) used to reanalyze data from the National Vietnam Veterans Readjustment Study (NVVRS; Kulka et al. 1990). The reanalysis showed that for male veterans, childhood antisocial behavior did not increase the likelihood of PTSD directly; it did, however, increase the likelihood indirectly by increasing the likelihood of war zone exposure, which in turn increased the likelihood of PTSD. There was no relationship between childhood antisocial behavior and exposure or PTSD in female veterans. It is unfortunate that the reanalysis did not include a measure of premilitary antisocial personality disorder. Nevertheless, if we assume that childhood behavior problems provide some indication of premilitary antisocial personality characteristics, the structural model may be interpreted as showing that pretraumatic antisocial personality is a risk factor for PTSD in that it increases the likelihood of traumatic exposure.

The observed association between PTSD and antisocial personality disorder cannot completely be explained as a function of pretraumatic personality, however. Additional data on male veterans implicate PTSD as a risk factor for adult antisocial behavior through pathways independent of the influence of pretraumatic antisocial behavior and its association with war zone exposure and PTSD. Barrett and colleagues (1996) found that PTSD was associated with increased likelihood of adult antisocial behavior even when they controlled for childhood behavior problems and war zone exposure. PTSD also was associated with increased likelihood of antisocial personality disorder when war zone exposure, but not childhood behavior problems, was controlled (presumably because of the necessary overlap between childhood problems and adult disorder). In combination, Barrett et al.'s and King et al.'s data on antisocial personality disorder and PTSD suggest a pattern of mutual influence over time.

With respect to the question of whether personality disorder is a risk factor for PTSD, it appears that antisocial personality could be, but that its relationship to PTSD is transactional: pretraumatic antisocial behavior may be a risk factor for PTSD, but PTSD in turn may lead to increases in antisocial behavior. There are insufficient data to permit conclusions about other personality disorders.

Specific Traits as Correlates of PTSD

In this subsection, we review empirical studies on the relationship between personality dimensions, or traits, and PTSD. The review is organized around three of the four trait dimensions in the hierarchical structure of personality traits proposed by Watson and colleagues (1994): *neuroticism,* or negative emotionality; *extraversion,* or positive emotionality; and *conscientiousness,* or constraint. (We did not find PTSD literature on the fourth dimension, *agreeableness.*) Table 9–1 illustrates how we have categorized traits according to these dimensions.

The terms *neuroticism, negative affectivity,* and *negative emotionality* all have been used to describe a broad personality dimension that has been proposed as a likely risk factor for PTSD because the dimension reflects sensitivity to negative stimuli (Clark et al. 1994). We use the term neuroticism here because it appears most often in the PTSD literature. Despite incomplete agreement on the particular component traits that are subsumed under this dimension, neuroticism is thought to consist of mood and nonmood components (Clark et al. 1994). In addition to neuroticism, components

Table 9–1. Categorization of personality traits examined in research on posttraumatic stress disorder

Personality dimension	Trait
Neuroticism/negative affectivity/ negative emotionality	Neuroticism
	Trait anxiety
	Hardiness
	Hostility
	Pessimism (attributional style, locus of control)
	Alexithymia
Extraversion/positive affectivity/ positive emotionality	Extraversion (introversion)
	Sensation seeking
Conscientiousness/constraint	Constraint/impulsivity
Agreeableness	None

Source. The dimensional model and rationale for classification are drawn from Clark et al. 1994 and Watson et al. 1994.

that have been explored in PTSD studies (and about which there seems to be generally good agreement as to their relationship to neuroticism) are trait anxiety, hardiness, hostility, and pessimism/attributional style. Our discussion of this dimension includes reference to alexithymia, given data about its relationship to neuroticism (Wise and Mann 1994), and locus of control, given its relationship to attributional style.

With the exception of Mayou and colleagues (1993), investigators who have studied clinical and nonclinical samples of combat and civilian trauma survivors have found that PTSD is positively correlated with neuroticism as measured by a variety of instruments (e.g., Breslau et al. 1991; Davidson et al. 1987; Hyer et al. 1994a; Kuhne et al. 1993; McFarlane 1988a; Weiss et al. 1995). Results of one longitudinal study suggest that higher levels of neuroticism are related to chronicity as well. McFarlane (1988b) found that individuals with chronic PTSD had significantly higher neuroticism scores than individuals with histories of only acute PTSD. Neuroticism was a better predictor of PTSD than level of trauma exposure in this study, accounting for an increasing proportion of the variance over time, while the contributions of trauma exposure variables progressively decreased. (Breslau and Davis [1992], who found that neuroticism was related to increased likelihood of both chronic and acute subtypes, did not report a direct comparison of differences in neuroticism between these subtypes.)

High trait anxiety also is related to PTSD in treatment-seeking and non–treatment-seeking adults and children (e.g., Blanchard et al. 1995; Lonigan et al. 1994; Sutker et al. 1991), although individuals with PTSD sometimes do not differ from psychiatric control subjects in terms of trait anxiety (e.g., Chemtob et al. 1994; Orr et al. 1990). Moreover, differences between PTSD and no-PTSD groups in trait anxiety scores have been found to be greater than differences in other indices, such as state anxiety, depression, and MMPI scale scores (Sutker et al. 1991). In one exception to the findings on trait anxiety, Shalev and colleagues (1996) found that individuals with PTSD 6 months after exposure to trauma differed in levels of state anxiety, but not trait anxiety, as assessed 1 week posttrauma.

Low hardiness has been linked to PTSD as well. L. A. King and colleagues (1998), in their reanalysis of the NVVRS dataset, used structural equation modeling to test a multivariate model of PTSD etiology that incorporated war zone stressors and postwar resilience and recovery variables, including hardiness. Low hardiness was a strong PTSD predictor relative to other resilience/recovery and war zone stressor variables examined. For both men and women, hardiness had a direct negative effect on PTSD, as well as a robust indirect effect, particularly through its association with more adequate social support. Sutker and colleagues (1995) performed double cross-validated discriminant function analyses and found that commitment, one of the three hardiness elements, was a consistent predictor of PTSD, accounting for 26% of the variance. The remaining two elements, sense of control and perception of change as challenging, also differentiated individuals with and without PTSD, though they failed to make any additional, substantive contributions to the discriminant function.

The interpretation of hostility as a risk factor for PTSD is especially difficult because irritability and anger are diagnostic indicators of the disorder. It is not surprising that many investigators have found that PTSD is associated with increased levels of hostility (e.g., Chemtob et al. 1994; Lasko et al. 1994) or lower levels of overcontrolled hostility (Silver and Salamone-Genovese 1991). Results of some studies suggest that PTSD may be differentially related to components of hostility. Lasko and colleagues (1994) found that individuals with PTSD scored significantly higher than individuals without PTSD on a measure of angry reactions but not on a measure of angry temperament. Similarly, Beckham and colleagues (1996) found that treatment-seeking PTSD-positive military veterans exhibited more paraverbal hostility (e.g., speaking in an irritated tone) than did non–treatment-seeking veterans without PTSD during administration of a behavioral hostility measure. However, no significant differences were noted with regard to levels of verbal hostility (e.g., direct verbal confrontation of interviewer).

Peterson and Seligman (1984) conceptualize pessimism in terms of attributional style, an individual's typical pattern of explanations for the events he or she has experienced. A pessimistic attributional style—one that is internal, global, and stable for negative events and the opposite for positive events—has been linked to depression (Peterson and Seligman 1984). Aspects of a pessimistic style are associated with PTSD in Vietnam veterans (McCormick et al. 1989), children (Wolfe et al. 1989), and college students (Falsetti and Resick 1995); additionally, in a study of disaster survivors, a positive attributional style was linked to increased support, which in turn was linked to decreased PTSD (Joseph et al. 1993a). In the one study to report contradictory results, Mikulincer and Solomon (1988) found that increases in PTSD symptoms over a 1-year interval were related to external and stable attributions for negative events and external attributions for positive events. The authors suggested that the unexpected pattern of findings may reflect a denial of responsibility among veterans with PTSD, but this explanation does not account for McCormick and colleagues' (1989) opposite findings with veterans. Joseph and colleagues (1993b) provide another reason for the discrepancy— a questionable measurement strategy used by Mikulincer and Solomon. Given the preponderance of the evidence, it is reasonable to conclude that PTSD is associated with a negative attributional style. Falsetti and Resick's (1995) data, however, raise questions about the specificity of the association between attributional style and PTSD relative to depression. These authors did not find any differences in attributional style between individuals with PTSD only, depression only, and both PTSD and depression.

Locus of control relates to the internality/externality component of attributional style. Investigations have consistently shown that PTSD is associated with scores indicating an external locus of control (e.g., Frye and Stockton 1982; Solomon et al. 1988; Weiss et al. 1995). Longitudinal data indicate that shifts toward internal locus of control are correlated with decreases in PTSD symptoms (Solomon et al. 1988). One interesting study showed that locus of control and PTSD were correlated only for soldiers who experienced an acute stress reaction under conditions of low battle intensity and not for those whose acute reaction occurred under conditions of high battle intensity (Solomon et al. 1989).

The data on PTSD and locus of control may seem to contradict the data linking PTSD with an attributional style that is characterized by internal attributions. When interpreting these seemingly contradictory findings, it is important to remember that a pessimistic attributional style involves making internal attributions for negative events and external attributions for positive events. As it turns out, the scale used in all of the investigations of PTSD and locus of control, Rotter's I-E scale (Rotter 1966), appears to measure locus of control for *positive* events (Brewin and Shapiro 1984). Thus, relatively external scores on this scale indicate perceptions of not being able to control the occurrence of desired outcomes.

Two studies have examined alexithymia in relation to PTSD. Zeitlin and colleagues (1993) found that alexithymia was positively related to degree of trauma exposure (i.e., number of assaults experienced), but they failed to find differences between rape victims with and without PTSD in degree of alexithymia. The failure to find a difference between PTSD and no-PTSD groups may have been not only because of the small sample size in this study but also because 8 of the 12 no-PTSD rape victims had a lifetime history of PTSD, even though they did not meet the criteria of this disorder at the time of assessment. In contrast, Yehuda and colleagues (1997) reported that PTSD and no-PTSD groups of non–treatment-seeking Holocaust survivors did not differ in amount of trauma exposure and that the PTSD group had relatively higher alexithymia scores. Not surprisingly, alexithymia was found to be most strongly related to the avoidance and hyperarousal symptoms of PTSD. This study is particularly noteworthy for its use of standardized diagnostic measures and its attention to potential confounding variables. With regard to the latter, individuals with concurrent Axis I disorders previously found to be associated with alexithymia were excluded from the subject pool.

Extraversion is a personality dimension that has been hypothesized by Clark and colleagues (1994) to be specific for depression, as compared with neuroticism, which is more broadly related to distress disorders. Individuals high in extraversion (the term used in the PTSD literature) or positive affectivity (a term often used in the personality literature) would be expected to display characteristics such as gregariousness, leadership, enjoying being the center of attention, cheerfulness, and seeking out stimulating experiences (Watson et al. 1994).

Extraversion has been linked to lower levels of PTSD in several studies, although the association seems to be less robust than the association between PTSD and neuroticism. Davidson and colleagues (1987) reported that World War II/Korean conflict veterans with PTSD were significantly more introverted than the age-matched nonpsychiatric control subjects, including both combat and noncombat veterans. The older veterans with PTSD also were more introverted than the Vietnam veterans with PTSD. Based on retrospective assessments, McFarlane (1988a, 1988b) found that Australian firefighters with PTSD were more introverted before the trauma than were their nonaffected counterparts. However, overall results indicated that extraversion played a much less prominent role than neuroticism in the longitudinal course of the disorder. Similarly, Kuhne and colleagues (1993), comparing groups of veterans with and without PTSD who were seeking treatment for substance abuse, found a much larger difference in neuroticism than in extraversion; the lower extraversion scores in the PTSD group were statistically significant, but not when the Bonferroni adjustment was made.

In contrast to their findings on neuroticism, Breslau and colleagues' (1991) findings on extraversion failed to show an association with PTSD. Hyer and co-workers (1994a) also found that among individuals with PTSD, symptom severity was correlated with neuroticism but not with extraversion. Reconciling these two studies with the data linking PTSD and introversion is complicated by the finding that in Breslau et al.'s sample, extraversion was related to increased likelihood of traumatic exposure (Breslau et al. 1991, 1995). If anything, the relationship between extraversion and exposure on the one hand and exposure and PTSD on the other should lead to extraversion's being related to PTSD, although indirectly, through exposure.

Results on sensation seeking, another component trait of extraversion, in relation to PTSD also are difficult to interpret. Sensation seeking has been linked to both favorable and unfavorable

PTSD outcomes. PTSD was unrelated to a global measure of sensation seeking in two studies (Orr et al. 1990, 1993), but in one of these studies, Vietnam veterans with PTSD scored higher than anxious combat control subjects on subscales for experience seeking and boredom susceptibility and higher than healthy combat control subjects on boredom susceptibility (Orr et al. 1990). Higher scores on the same global measure of sensation seeking used in Orr et al.'s studies were unrelated to PTSD symptoms in Israeli combat veterans (Solomon et al. 1995). However, scores on the global measure were related to lower PTSD symptoms among former POWs, a pattern of findings that led the authors to suggest that sensation seeking may function as a buffering variable under conditions of high stress.

Individuals high on the personality dimension of conscientiousness, or constraint, plan carefully before acting, are reliable and self-disciplined, have high achievement aspirations, respect authority, and avoid risky or dangerous situations (Watson et al. 1994). Only a few studies of Vietnam veteran samples have examined how PTSD relates to this dimension, and the majority of data show little relationship. In one study (Kuhne et al. 1993), groups of veterans with PTSD and those without PTSD did not differ in constraint, but the PTSD group had higher impulsivity scores (although not when Bonferroni adjustment was made). In another study, there were no differences in behavioral indicators of impulsivity between PTSD, psychiatric, and healthy combat groups (Chemtob et al. 1994). In a third study, constraint was correlated with PTSD symptoms on only one of the four PTSD assessment instruments used by the investigators (Hyer et al. 1994a).

Findings from cross-sectional studies of relationships between PTSD and specific traits show clear associations of this disorder with neuroticism and its components. The evidence regarding extraversion and constraint is equivocal and shows a lack of uniformity in how the component traits of these dimensions relate to PTSD. The data do not permit strong inferences about the extent to which the observed associations are unique to PTSD versus more general to other psychiatric disorders. The data also do not permit strong inferences about the extent to which these associations reflect the influence of PTSD on personality. Neuroticism has been suggested not just as an outcome but also as a vulnerability factor for depression (Clark et al. 1994); the same is likely true for PTSD.

Studies With Antecedent Personality Measures

Only a few studies have examined the association between personality and PTSD with measures of personality that were obtained prior to traumatic exposure. All of these studies assessed combat-related PTSD in male military veterans.

Card (1983) used archival data from Project TALENT to examine the relationship between personality traits at age 15 years and PTSD assessed at age 36 in a group of Vietnam veterans. Of 10 personality variables assessed in adolescence, only low self-confidence was associated with higher PTSD symptoms at age 36. The lack of association between PTSD and other variables is difficult to interpret because of the restricted content validity of the PTSD scale, which was constructed post hoc from items that did not fully capture diagnostic criteria for the disorder (e.g., there were no items assessing intrusive memories, flashbacks, or avoidance of traumatic reminders). (The limitations of the scale are perhaps best indicated by the actual difference of 3 points between Vietnam-theater and Vietnam-era veterans, despite a theoretical range of 16 to 80.)

Lee and colleagues (1995) presented data based on a longitudinal assessment of World War II combat veterans who were first studied while undergraduates at Harvard University. Like Card, Lee et al. used a PTSD measure that was constructed post hoc, but the latter's measure appears to have adequate content validity. Psychological soundness in college, a general measure of emotional/psychological difficulties, was not related to PTSD symptoms assessed immediately after the war. Also, psychological defenses from ages 20 to 47 and poor psychosocial adjustment from ages 30 to 44, which might be loosely interpreted as reflecting personality variables, were not related to PTSD symptoms at age 65 (but they were related to neuroticism at age 65).

Schnurr and colleagues (1993) examined the relationship between personality and PTSD by reviewing college MMPI profiles of Vietnam combat and Vietnam-era veterans from the Dartmouth College classes of 1967 and 1968. Group means on the MMPI scales were all within normal limits. The Structured Clinical Interview for DSM-III-R (Spitzer et al. 1987) was used to assess lifetime PTSD, as well as to subdivide participants according to whether they met full or subthreshold criteria for the disorder or only had a lifetime history of some PTSD symptoms. In contrast to the studies discussed above, this study found that premilitary personality scores were related to PTSD symptomatology. Hypochondriasis, Psychopathic Deviate, Masculinity–Femininity, and Paranoia scale scores all predicted lifetime PTSD symptoms (full, subthreshold, or symptoms), with Psychopathic Deviate and Masculinity–Femininity being the strongest predictors. Furthermore, Social Introversion was found to be the best predictor of PTSD subclassification, although depression and hypomania also distinguished among PTSD subgroups. There was a nonlinear relationship between PTSD subgroup and Social Introversion. Veterans who developed only PTSD symptoms were more introverted than veterans who developed either full PTSD or subthreshold PTSD, but those in the full group were more introverted than those in the subthreshold group. Control for amount of combat exposure failed to have a significant impact on any of the findings.

Schnurr et al. (1993) suggested that, given the normal range of mean MMPI scale scores, combat-related PTSD symptomatology is positively associated with the following personality features (organized in terms of the three broad personality dimensions discussed above): dissatisfaction, gloominess, irritability (neuroticism); shyness, withdrawal (extraversion); and impulsivity, inhibition, conscientiousness (constraint). Normal-range social introversion scores, which distinguished the PTSD subgroups, may reflect characteristics of extraversion and constraint: shyness, withdrawal, and inhibition, as well as impulse-control problems and extraversion.

These findings thus implicate not just neuroticism but also extraversion and constraint in the etiology of PTSD. Reconciling these findings with the null results of Card (1983) and Lee et al.

(1995), one could speculate that the use of validated measures of both PTSD and personality by Schnurr et al. (1993) provided a more sensitive test of the relationship between personality and PTSD than was provided in the other two studies. Of course, replication of these results in future studies with pretraumatic personality measures is critically needed. This one study, however, lends support to the view that personality is a true risk factor for PTSD and not merely a risk marker or outcome of the disorder.

Conclusion

Despite the lack of data that permit strong inferences about the relationship between antecedent personality factors and the development of PTSD, some conclusions are possible.

First, there is ample evidence linking personality and PTSD. The most striking finding is that neuroticism and its component traits are consistently associated with PTSD. Virtually all of the evidence is cross-sectional and retrospective, but some is not.

Second, personality could function as a risk factor for PTSD. We presented a model of how personality could influence reactions to trauma (Mischel and Shoda 1995) and discussed several mediating factors, including an individual's immediate reactions to a stressor, cognitive processing of the stressor, and ability to enlist social support for help in dealing with the stressor or its aftermath. In addition to influencing how individuals react to traumatic events, personality may affect the risk of PTSD by influencing risk of exposure to traumatic events. Breslau and colleagues (1995) followed a sample of young adults for 3 years and found that neuroticism and extraversion measured at the beginning of the study were associated with increased risk of traumatic exposure during the observation period, even when the effects of traumatic exposure prior to the study and other variables were controlled. Neuroticism and extraversion also were associated with increased risk of exposure in cross-sectional analyses to predict lifetime exposure (Breslau et al. 1991, 1995).

So, even though virtually all of the evidence comes from cross-sectional studies that are inherently ambiguous with regard to issues of causality, we believe it is likely that personality plays a role in the etiology of PTSD—a conclusion that has significant implications for both research and practice. We will never fully understand the etiology of PTSD if we fail to correctly specify the way that pretraumatic factors influence reactions to trauma. We also will never be able to predict PTSD very well if we sweep the variation in PTSD prevalence due to pretraumatic variables into an error term. Poor predictive power, in turn, will hinder efforts at either primary or secondary prevention.

However, more is needed than simply recognizing and investigating the role played by pretraumatic personality and other pretraumatic variables in the development of PTSD. Because of its correlational nature, this research should be conducted with increased rigor and should use measures collected prior to traumatization whenever possible—for example, by focusing on cohorts such as military personnel who have a high likelihood of traumatic exposure. Greater attention to the distinction between the development of PTSD and its maintenance is especially important; we have virtually no information about how personality factors relate to recovery. Multiple posttraumatic assessments of both personality and PTSD will further our understanding of how these variables relate to one another over time. Lastly, research is needed to bridge our understanding of personality and other risk factors for PTSD to diathesis-stress models of depression and other psychiatric disorders. It would be helpful to know whether specific personality constructs operate similarly or differently in affecting risk of PTSD versus other disorders. For example, neuroticism, implicated herein as a risk factor for PTSD, is a likely risk factor for depression and other anxiety disorders (Clark et al. 1994).

Perhaps the greatest challenge for future research is the need to specify *how* personality operates as a risk factor—that is, how does neuroticism or any other aspect of personality influence the processing of traumatic material? The model of personality offered by Mischel and Shoda (1995) offers much promise in this regard, and more than is offered by traditional trait-behavior theory. At present, data on the cognitive and affective correlates of PTSD do not conclusively demonstrate that pretraumatic differences in cognitive-affective units are responsible for the development of PTSD in traumatized individuals. What is clear, though, is that individuals with and without PTSD differ in terms of all five types of cognitive-affective units. We offer the following examples.

With respect to *encodings*, PTSD is correlated with negative views of self and others (Dutton et al. 1994). *Expectancies and beliefs* also vary as a function of one's PTSD status. Janoff-Bulman (1992) has proposed that trauma violates basic assumptions about one's safety, the fairness of the world, and the predictability of aversive events. *Affects*, especially physiological reactions, differ as well (Prins et al. 1995). Shalev and colleagues (1996) found that peritraumatic dissociation measured in the week after a traumatic event predicted PTSD at 6 months; peritraumatic dissociation, in turn, has been shown to be related to the personality constructs of shyness and inhibition (Marmar et al. 1996). Although little is known about the *goals and values* associated with PTSD, a sense of foreshortened future—a diminished future orientation—is one of the symptom criteria for PTSD. In contrast, much more is known about PTSD and coping strategies, which encompass *competencies and self-regulatory plans*. Relative to individuals without PTSD, those with PTSD are more likely to use nonoptimal strategies such as emotion-focused and avoidant coping (e.g., Valentiner et al. 1996). Interesting evidence of relationships among coping strategies and personality characteristics comes from a study of PTSD patients in whom unique associations between particular strategies and personality traits were found (Hyer et al. 1996). For example, although antisocial and passive-aggressive characteristics were positively correlated with confrontive coping, antisocial characteristics were negatively correlated with escape-avoidance strategies, and passive-aggressive characteristics were positively associated with escape-avoidance.

The cross-sectional nature of these examples and of virtually all of the relevant data prevents us from knowing to what extent the differences associated with PTSD are outcomes rather than predisposing variables. Indeed, it is not just plausible but also likely that cognitive affective units and their organization are altered by the development of PTSD. Nevertheless, pretraumatic differences in cognitive affective units and their organization could function within the theoretical framework provided by Mischel and Shoda (1995) to explain how personality could affect reactions to trauma. It would be helpful if future research were to employ measurement strategies that operationalize cognitive affective units in addition to, or even rather than, traditional trait measures.

Our conclusions about the role of personality in the etiology of PTSD may be viewed in the broader context of diathesis-stress models for psychiatric disorders (e.g., Meehl 1962). For example, a recent review of the literature on personality as diathesis for depression begins with the assertion, "Most people do not become clinically depressed even when confronted with ostensibly serious stressors" (Coyne and Whiffen 1995, p. 358). If we substituted the words "develop PTSD" for "become clinically depressed" and "traumatic" for "ostensibly serious," we would have something akin to the premise of this chapter. Coyne and Whiffen (1995) state, "*Diathesis-stress* models of depression are widely seen as a significant advance over the simplistic assumption that all persons are equally vulnerable to depression" (p. 358, emphasis in original). Is the same true for PTSD? During the 1980s, the answer probably would have been a relatively strong "no." Today—many data later—we hope the answer would be at least a modest "yes."

References

Ahlbom A, Norell S: Introduction to Modern Epidemiology. Chestnut Hill, MA, Epidemiology Resources, 1990

American Psychiatric Association: Diagnostic and Statistical Manual of Mental Disorders, 3rd Edition. Washington, DC, American Psychiatric Association, 1980

American Psychiatric Association: Diagnostic and Statistical Manual of Mental Disorders, 4th Edition. Washington, DC, American Psychiatric Association, 1994

Barrett DH, Resnick HS, Foy DW, et al: Combat exposure and adult psychosocial adjustment among U.S. Army veterans serving in Vietnam, 1965–1971. J Abnorm Psychol 105:575–581, 1996

Beckham JC, Roodman AA, Barefoot JC, et al: Interpersonal and self-reported hostility among combat veterans with and without posttraumatic stress disorder. J Trauma Stress 9:335–342, 1996

Blanchard EB, Hickling EJ, Taylor AE, et al: Psychiatric morbidity associated with motor vehicle accidents. J Nerv Ment Dis 183:495–504, 1995

Breslau N, Davis GC: Posttraumatic stress disorder in an urban population of young adults: risk factors for chronicity. Am J Psychiatry 149: 671–675, 1992

Breslau N, Davis GC, Andreski P, et al: Traumatic events and post-traumatic stress disorder in an urban population of young adults. Arch Gen Psychiatry 48:216–222, 1991

Breslau N, Davis GC, Andreski P: Risk factors for PTSD-related traumatic events: a prospective analysis. Am J Psychiatry 152:529–535, 1995

Brewin CR, Shapiro DA: Beyond locus of control: attributions of responsibility for positive and negative outcomes. Br J Psychol 75:43–49, 1984

Brill NQ, Beebe GW: A Follow-up Study of War Neuroses. Washington, DC, Veterans Administration, 1955

Butcher JN, Williams CL: Essentials of MMPI-2 and MMPI-A Interpretation. Minneapolis, University of Minnesota Press, 1992

Card JJ: Lives After Vietnam: The Personal Impact of Military Service. Lexington, MA, Lexington Books, 1983

Chemtob CM, Hamada RS, Roitblat HL, et al: Anger, impulsivity, and anger control in combat-related posttraumatic stress disorder. J Consult Clin Psychol 62:827–832, 1994

Clark LA, Watson D, Mineka S: Temperament, personality, and the mood and anxiety disorders. J Abnorm Psychol 103:103–116, 1994

Cook TD, Campbell DT: Quasi-Experimentation. Chicago, IL, Rand McNally, 1979

Coyne JC, Whiffen VE: Issues in personality as diathesis for depression: the case of sociotrophy-dependency and autonomy-self-criticism. Psychol Bull 118:358–378, 1995

Davidson J, Kudler H, Smith R: Personality in chronic post-traumatic stress disorder: a study of the Eysenck Inventory. J Anxiety Disord 1:295–300, 1987

Davis S (ed): Connectionism: Theory and Practice. New York, Oxford University Press, 1992

Dutton MA, Burghardt KJ, Perrin SG, et al: Battered women's cognitive schemata. J Trauma Stress 7:237–255, 1994

Engdahl BE, Speed N, Eberly RE, et al: Comorbidity of psychiatric disorders and personality profiles of American World War II prisoners of war. J Nerv Ment Dis 179:181–187, 1991

Falsetti SA, Resick PA: Causal attributions, depression, and posttraumatic stress disorder in victims of crime. J Appl Soc Psychol 25: 1027–1042, 1995

Foa EB, Steketee G, Rothbaum BO: Behavioral/cognitive conceptualizations of posttraumatic stress disorder. Behavior Therapy 20:155–176, 1989

Foy DW, Sipprelle RC, Rueger DB, et al: Etiology of posttraumatic stress disorder in Vietnam veterans: analysis of premilitary, military, and combat exposure influences. J Consult Clin Psychol 52:79–87, 1984

Frederick CJ: Children traumatized by catastrophic situations, in Posttraumatic Stress Disorder in Children. Edited by Eth S, Pynoos RS. Washington, DC, American Psychiatric Association, 1985, pp 71–99

Friedman MJ, Rosenheck RA: PTSD as a persistent mental illness, in Handbook for the Treatment of the Seriously Mentally Ill. Edited by Soreff SM. Seattle, WA, Hogrefe & Huber, 1996, pp 369–389

Frye JS, Stockton RA: Discriminant analysis of posttraumatic stress disorder among a group of Vietnam veterans. Am J Psychiatry 139:52–56, 1982

Gaston L, Brunet A, Koszycki D, et al: MMPI profiles of acute and chronic PTSD in a civilian sample. J Trauma Stress 9:817–832, 1996

Goldberg LR: An alternative "description of personality": the Big-Five factor structure. J Pers Soc Psychol 59:1216–1229, 1990

Green BL, Grace MC, Lindy JD, et al: Risk factors for PTSD and other diagnoses in a general sample of Vietnam veterans. Am J Psychiatry 147:729–733, 1990

Hathaway SR, McKinley JC: Minnesota Multiphasic Personality Inventory Manual. New York, Psychological Corporation, 1967

Helzer JE, Robins LN, McEvoy L: Post-traumatic stress disorder in the general population: findings of the Epidemiologic Catchment Area Survey. N Engl J Med 317:1630–1634, 1987

Hyer L, Woods MG, Boudewyns PA, et al: MCMI and 16-PF with Vietnam veterans: profiles and concurrent validation of MCMI. Journal of Personality Disorders 4:391–401, 1990

Hyer L, Braswell L, Albrecht W, et al: Relationship of NEO-PI to personality styles and severity of trauma in chronic PTSD victims. J Clin Psychol 50:699–707, 1994a

Hyer L, Davis H, Albrecht W, et al: Cluster analysis of MCMI and MCMI-II on chronic PTSD victims. J Clin Psychol 50:502–515, 1994b

Hyer L, McCranie EW, Boudewyns PA, et al: Modes of long-term coping with trauma memories: relative use and associations with personality among Vietnam veterans with chronic PTSD. J Trauma Stress 9:299–316, 1996

Janoff-Bulman R: Shattered Assumptions: Towards a New Psychology of Trauma. New York, Free Press, 1992

Joseph S, Brewin CR, Yule W, et al: Causal attributions and posttraumatic stress in adolescents. J Child Psychol Psychiatry 34:247–253, 1993a

Joseph S, Yule W, Williams R: Post-traumatic stress: attributional aspects. J Trauma Stress 6:501–513, 1993b

Keane TM, Malloy PF, Fairbank JA: Empirical development of an MMPI subscale for the assessment of combat-related posttraumatic stress disorder. J Consult Clin Psychol 52:888–891, 1984

Kessler RC, Sonnega A, Bromet E, et al: Posttraumatic stress disorder in the National Comorbidity Survey. Arch Gen Psychiatry 52:1048–1060, 1995

King DW, King LA, Foy DW, et al: Prewar factors in combat-related posttraumatic stress disorder: structural equation modeling with a national sample of female and male Vietnam veterans. J Consult Clin Psychol 64:520–531, 1996

King LA, King DW, Fairbank JA, et al: Resilience/recovery factors in posttraumatic stress disorder among male and female Vietnam veterans: hardiness, postwar social support, and additional stressful life events. J Pers Soc Psychol 74:420–434, 1998

Kluznik JC, Speed N, Van Valkenburg C, et al: Forty-year follow-up of United States prisoners of war. Am J Psychiatry 143:1443–1446, 1986

Koretzky MB, Peck AH: Validation and cross-validation of the PTSD subscale of the MMPI with civilian trauma victims. J Clin Psychol 46:296–300, 1990

Kuhne A, Orr SP, Baraga E: Psychometric evaluation of post-traumatic stress disorder: the Multidimensional Personality Questionnaire as an adjunct to the MMPI. J Clin Psychol 49:218–225, 1993

Kulka RA, Schlenger WE, Fairbank JA, et al: Trauma and the Vietnam War Generation. New York, Brunner/Mazel, 1990

Lasko NB, Gurvits TV, Kuhne AA, et al: Aggression and its correlates in Vietnam veterans with and without chronic posttraumatic stress disorder. Compr Psychiatry 35:373–381, 1994

Lee KA, Vaillant GE, Torrey WC, et al: A 50-year prospective study of the psychological sequelae of World War II combat. Am J Psychiatry 152: 516–522, 1995

Lindzey G, Hall CS, Manosevitz M: Theories of Personality: Primary Sources and Research. Malabar, FL, Robert E Krieger, 1988

Lonigan CJ, Shannon MP, Taylor CM, et al: Children exposed to disaster, II: risk factors for the development of post-traumatic symptomatology. J Am Acad Child Adolesc Psychiatry 33:94–105, 1994

Marmar CR, Weiss DS, Metzler TJ, et al: Characteristics of emergency services personnel related to peritraumatic dissociation during critical incident exposure. Am J Psychiatry 153(suppl):94–102, 1996

Mayou R, Bryant B, Duthie R: Psychiatric consequences of road traffic accidents. BMJ 307:647–651, 1993

McCormick RA, Taber JI, Kruedelback N: The relationship between attributional style and post-traumatic stress disorder in addicted patients. J Trauma Stress 2:477–487, 1989

McCrae RR, Costa PT: Toward a new generation of personality theories: theoretical contexts for the five-factor model, in The Five-Factor Model of Personality: Theoretical Perspectives. Edited by Wiggins JS. New York, Guilford, 1996, pp 51–87

McFarlane AC: The aetiology of post-traumatic stress disorders following a natural disaster. Br J Psychiatry 152:116–121, 1988a

McFarlane AC: The longitudinal course of posttraumatic morbidity: the range of outcomes and their predictors. J Nerv Ment Dis 176:30–39, 1988b

Meehl PE: Schizotaxia, schizotypy, schizophrenia. Am Psychol 17: 827–838, 1962

Mikulincer M, Solomon Z: Attributional style and combat-related posttraumatic stress disorder. J Abnorm Psychol 97:308–313, 1988

Millon T: Manual for the MCMI-II. Minneapolis, MN, National Computer Systems, 1987

Mischel W, Shoda Y: A cognitive-affective system theory of personality: reconceptualizing situations, dispositions, dynamics, and invariance in personality structure. Psychol Rev 102:246–268, 1995

Orr SP, Clairborn JM, Altman B, et al: Psychometric profile of post-traumatic stress disorder, anxious, and healthy Vietnam veterans: correlations with psychophysiologic responses. J Consult Clin Psychol 58:329–335, 1990

Orr SP, Pitman RK, Lasko NB, et al: Psychophysiological assessment of posttraumatic stress disorder imagery in World War II and Korean combat veterans. J Abnorm Psychol 102:152–159, 1993

Peterson C, Seligman MEP: Causal explanations as a risk factor for depression: theory and evidence. Psychol Rev 91:96–103, 1984

Prins A, Kaloupek DG, Keane TM: Psychophysiological evidence for autonomic arousal and startle in traumatized adult populations, in Neurobiological and Clinical Consequences of Stress: From Normal Adaptation to Post-traumatic Stress Disorder. Edited by Friedman MJ, Charney DS, Deutch AY. Philadelphia, PA, Lippincott–Raven, 1995, pp 291–314

Resnick HS, Foy DW, Donahoe CP, et al: Antisocial behavior and post-traumatic stress disorder in Vietnam veterans. J Clin Psychol 45: 860–866, 1989

Robert JA, Ryan JJ, McEntyre WL, et al: MCMI characteristics of DSM-III posttraumatic stress disorder in Vietnam veterans. J Pers Assess 49: 226–230, 1985

Rotter JB: Generalized expectancies for internal versus external control of reinforcement. Psychological Monographs 80:1–28, 1966

Schnurr PP, Friedman MJ, Rosenberg SD: Premilitary MMPI scores as predictors of combat-related PTSD symptoms. Am J Psychiatry 150: 479–483, 1993

Shalev AY, Peri T, Canetti L, et al: Predictors of PTSD in injured trauma survivors: a prospective study. Am J Psychiatry 153:219–225, 1996

Silver SM, Salamone-Genovese L: A study of the MMPI clinical and research scales for post-traumatic stress disorder diagnostic utility. J Trauma Stress 4:533–548, 1991

Solomon Z, Mikulincer M, Avitzur E: Coping, locus of control, social support, and combat-related posttraumatic stress disorder: a prospective study. J Pers Soc Psychol 55:279–285, 1988

Solomon Z, Mikulincer M, Benbenishty R: Locus of control and combat-related post-traumatic stress disorder: the intervening role of battle intensity, threat appraisal and coping. Br J Clin Psychol 28:131–144, 1989

Solomon Z, Ginzburg K, Neria Y, et al: Coping with war captivity: the role of sensation-seeking. European Journal of Personality 9:57–70, 1995

Spitzer RL, Williams JBW, Gibbon M: Structured Clinical Interview for DSM-III-R, Version NP-V. New York, New York State Psychiatric Institute, Biometrics Research, 1987

Sutker PB, Bugg F, Allain AN: Psychometric prediction of PTSD among POW survivors. Psychological Assessment 3:105–110, 1991

Sutker PB, Davis JM, Uddo M, et al: War zone stress, personal resources, and PTSD in Persian Gulf War returnees. J Abnorm Psychol 104:444–452, 1995

Valentiner DP, Foa EB, Riggs DS, et al: Coping strategies and posttraumatic stress disorder in female victims of sexual and nonsexual assault. J Abnorm Psychol 105:455–458, 1996

Watson D, Clark LA: Introduction to "Special Issue on Personality and Pathology." J Abnorm Psychol 103:3–5, 1994

Watson D, Clark LA, Harkness AR: Structures of personality and their relevance to psychopathology. J Abnorm Psychol 103:18–31, 1994

Weiss DS, Marmar CR, Metzler TJ, et al: Predicting symptomatic distress in emergency services personnel. J Consult Clin Psychol 63:361–368, 1995

Wilson JP, Krauss GE: Predicting post-traumatic stress disorders among Vietnam veterans, in Post-Traumatic Stress Disorder and the War Veteran Patient. Edited by Kelly WE. New York, Brunner/Mazel, 1985, pp 102–147

Wise TN, Mann LS: The relationship between somatosensory amplification, alexithymia, and neuroticism. J Psychosom Res 38:515–521, 1994

Wolfe VV, Gentile C, Wolfe DA: The impact of sexual abuse on children: a PTSD formulation. Behavior Therapy 20:215–228, 1989

Yehuda R, Steiner A, Kahana B, et al: Alexithymia in Holocaust survivors with and without PTSD. J Trauma Stress 10:93–100, 1997

Yehuda R, McFarlane AC: Conflict between current knowledge about posttraumatic stress disorder and its original conceptual basis. Am J Psychiatry 152:1705–1713, 1995

Zeitlin SB, McNally RJ, Cassiday KL: Alexithymia in victims of sexual assault: an effect of repeated traumatization? Am J Psychiatry 150:661–663, 1993

Chapter 10

Risk Factors for PTSD: Reflections and Recommendations

Matthew J. Friedman, M.D., Ph.D.

This book, *Risk Factors for Postraumatic Stress Disorder*, edited by Rachel Yehuda, celebrates our growing appreciation of the many complex factors that make some individuals more vulnerable and others more resistant to PTSD following exposure to catastrophic stress. It shows just how far we have progressed from the original PTSD construct, that in DSM-III (American Psychiatric Association 1980), which minimized internal individual differences while emphasizing the magnitude and characteristics of the external stressor. The general belief at that time was that the importance of personal, genetic, experiential, adaptive, psychological, and psychobiological factors was dwarfed by the titanic impact of the external stressor itself. This belief was reinforced by many studies showing that there was a dose-response relationship between exposure to trauma and the development of PTSD. "But for the grace of God," the DSM-III seemed to say, anyone might be in the wrong place at the wrong time—anyone might develop PTSD.

Constructs such as "traumatic neurosis" that, in effect, blamed the victim for some sort of constitutional deficiency if he or she succumbed to posttraumatic distress were repudiated by the DSM-III. Indeed, one of the profound advantages of the original PTSD construct was that it was, arguably, the first Axis I disorder to be completely destigmatized. If everyone was at equal risk for PTSD, then we were all operating on a level psychological playing field. As the chapters in this book attest, however, such an egalitarian pretraumatic null hypothesis can no longer be sustained.

While reviewing the exciting chapters in this book, I had two personal reflections that had not occurred to me in many years. The first was intensely personal, while the second was the kind of obscure literature citation that is generally expected in discussions of this sort.

During World War II, my father was senior medical officer at a large military induction center in West Virginia. Although I could not have been more than 3 or 4 years old at the time, I recall a dinnertime conversation in which he mentioned that many military potential inductees had been rejected because of a history of enuresis. No doubt, the vividness of my own or my younger brother's struggle for complete bladder control at that impressionable age made this one of the few parental remarks I have retained from that early period. It must have come as quite a shock at the time for me to realize that I had better not wet the bed again if I ever hoped to command an aircraft carrier. From the perspective of this book, however, my father's remark reflects the military's long-standing effort to identify risk factors for shell shock or war neurosis so that vulnerable individuals could be identified before they were inducted into the armed forces. Davidson and Connor, in Chapter 4, review many of the early publications that illustrate how psychiatric attention was focused on constitutional-hereditary factors such as a personal or family history of nervousness, alcoholism, epilepsy, or insanity during both World Wars. With respect to the list of exclusionary criteria that guided my father and his fellow physicians as they examined and interviewed thousands of potential recruits at military induction centers throughout the United States, I was fascinated to learn from Orr and Pitman in Chapter 6 that a history of enuresis was reported more frequently by Vietnam veterans with PTSD than by those without.

My second recollection is of a modest study Suzanne Griffin and I (Griffin and Friedman 1986) carried out to detect depressive symptomatology among cardiovascular patients receiving the beta-adrenergic antagonist propranolol for angina, hypertension, or cardiac arrhythmia. There were two findings. Among cardiovascular patients who had neither a personal nor a family history of depression, we found a significant correlation between the dose of propranolol and the magnitude of depression scores on the Hamilton Depression Scale. There was no such relationship, however, for patients with a personal or family history of depression. Many such patients had very high depression scores, even though they had been prescribed relatively low doses of propranolol. We interpreted this second finding as consistent with a stress-diathesis model of depression. We argued that patients with a positive history were more vulnerable to the depressogenic actions of propranolol, whereas patients with a negative depressive history were more likely to exhibit a dose-response relationship. Like most studies reported in this book, ours was based on cross-sectional data. We had no way of knowing predrug depression levels, nor were we able to monitor any of these patients longitudinally. Despite these methodological weaknesses, our interpretation was both reasonable and consistent with prevailing beliefs about depression, although it certainly was not conclusive.

The Need for Longitudinal Research

Although most of the studies reported throughout this book are much more sophisticated and methodologically sound than the small study described in the previous section, they are generally based on cross-sectional data. Without pretraumatic measurement of variables of interest, it is impossible to separate cause from effect. Were abnormalities that distinguish PTSD individuals from others present before the trauma? Did they appear only after the trauma? Are they bona fide risk factors or risk indicators for PTSD? Are they direct or indirect predictors of PTSD?

We have learned a great deal from cross-sectional correlations, epidemiological data, and genetic studies. As Harvey and Yehuda emphasize in Chapter 1, longitudinal research is needed. They point out that PTSD is an ideal disorder to study with a longitudinal design because the traumatic stressor is discrete and observable. They suggest that we study either populations at risk because of predictable occupational hazards (e.g., military, police, emergency medical personnel) or populations with risk factors for PTSD, as determined by current data and theories and summarized in the present volume (e.g., prior exposure, family history, neurocognitive deficiency, psychophysiological vulnerability, personality factors). It is noteworthy that several nations currently engaged in United Nations (UN)/NATO peacekeeping activities are supporting research of this nature. During the 1996 European Conference on Traumatic Stress held in Maastricht, The Netherlands, researchers from different countries reported on their attempts to identify predictors of PTSD among military personnel who had been stationed in Cambodia, South Lebanon, the Persian Gulf, Somalia, and Bosnia. They have studied theoretical constructs such as Antonovsky's "sense of coherence," "hardiness," and the importance of positive versus negative appraisals as predictors of PTSD. The value of such work would be magnified greatly if UN/NATO troops could be followed longitudinally after predeployment evaluations have been carried out. Indeed, the United States government has begun to consider routine predeployment measurement of variables that might have a bearing on postdeployment medical and mental health outcomes. Such a programmatic initiative would constitute a major advance in our efforts to understand risk factors for PTSD and other adverse posttraumatic outcomes.

It will be difficult enough to improve our understanding about risk factors for PTSD. As we do so, we must recognize that most people exposed to trauma do not develop PTSD. Even if we restrict our analysis to worst-case scenarios, the "most upsetting traumas" surveyed by Kessler and associates in the National Comorbidity Survey (see Chapter 2), it is clear that the vast majority of American men and women never develop PTSD. Yehuda and McFarlane (1995) have argued that there is something fundamentally different about people who do and do not develop PTSD. Does this difference stem from genetic, experiential, neurocognitive, psychophysiological, or characterological factors, or from all of the above in a bewildering array of permutations? In addition to PTSD, should we start to pay closer attention to other potential adverse outcomes following exposure to traumatic events, such as other DSM-IV diagnoses (American Psychiatric Association 1994), medical illnesses, somatization, dissociation, or other idioms of distress that may emerge only in a cross-cultural context and may not conform to any DSM-IV nosologic category?

There is an implicit assumption in most of the current research on risk factors that people exposed to catastrophic stress who do not develop PTSD have coped successfully with their traumatic experience. Such an all-or-none categorical approach to this question may interfere with our opportunity to understand the subtle complexities of processes through which a terrifying experience is transformed into a stable psychiatric abnormality. As Schnurr and Vielhauer state in Chapter 9, it is not enough to know that certain personality factors predict PTSD; we must try to understand how personality might differentially affect an individual's response to trauma. Shalev provides, in Chapter 7, some of the most elegant theoretical, yet measurable, tools in this regard by identifying differences in psychophysiological response biases such as pretraumatic heightened reactivity, heightened conditionability, and/or impaired extinction as potential risk factors for PTSD. Such variables could be monitored longitudinally whether or not an individual develops, maintains, or recovers from PTSD.

The Complexity of PTSD

PTSD is a very complex disorder. We have proposed elsewhere that PTSD represents an abnormality in which the many psychobiological mechanisms that promote coping and adaptation have been overwhelmed by a catastrophic stress. We believe that the result is a shift from homeostasis to allostasis marked by alterations in many neurotransmitter/neurohormonal systems, and abnormalities in learning, memory, and information processing. People with PTSD tend to appraise the world as dangerous and have lost their ability to modify their behavior appropriately in response to changing environmental contingencies (Friedman et al. 1995).

Given the complexity of PTSD, there are many different pathways through which a particular risk factor might express itself. Kessler and associates' epidemiological findings show that female gender, less education, lower income, previous martial status, certain ethnic memberships, and certain pretraumatic psychiatric disorders are all risk factors for PTSD. These findings are fortified by Davidson and Connor's data showing that a family history of depression is a risk factor for PTSD (see Chapter 4) and by Yehuda's observations that children of Holocaust survivors appear to be at greater risk of developing PTSD than do an appropriate comparison group (see Chapter 5). Likewise, Orr and Pitman provide evidence that poorer intellectual ability and/or a compromised neurodevelopmental history constitute a neurocognitive risk factor for developing PTSD (see Chapter 6). Such information is certainly valuable for identifying populations at risk, planning intervention strategies, and informing public policy. They are, however, only a starting point for understanding the etiological significance of such risk factors. Genetic studies show that even after controlling for genetic factors that influence exposure to trauma, as True and Lyons point out in Chapter 3, "there is still a substantial genetic influence on how vulnerable an individual is to developing PTSD." True and Lyons speculate that genetically influenced personality characteristics may play a role both in the risk of trauma exposure and in vulnerability or resistance to PTSD. Psychobiological research shows that inherited or acquired abnormalities in hypothalamic-pituitary-adrenocortical function (see Chapter 5) or impaired ability to modulate physiological reactivity (see Chapter 7) represents still another important domain of risk factors for PTSD.

Schnurr and Vielhauer, in Chapter 9, take us through the next critical steps by invoking Mischel and Shoda's (1995) theory of a Cognitive-Affective Personality System to explain "processes underlying individual differences in cognitive, affective, and behavioral reactions to situations." According to this theory, there are five different domains of "cognitive-affective units." Abnormalities in any one (or in any combination) of such cognitive-affective units might be a risk factor for PTSD. For example, compromised *encoding* might affect information processing, learning, or memory; altered *expectancies and beliefs* might affect the appraisal process; altered *affects* would have an impact on emotional and physiological responses to events; and so forth. As noted by Schnurr and

Vielhauer, this theoretical approach lends itself very well to connectionist models of information processing and to influential clinical theoretical approaches such as Foa and colleagues' (1989) cognitive conceptualization of PTSD as the result of traumatically activated fear structures. The beauty of the heuristic approach proposed by Schnurr and Vielhauer is that it helps us formulate mechanisms through which a variety of different risk factors might operate on a variety of crucial mechanisms that mediate vulnerability or resistance to PTSD.

Shalev provides operational definitions for hypothesized psychophysiological mechanisms that may mediate vulnerability or resistance to PTSD (see Chapter 7). This elegant approach generates testable predictions that could be monitored in longitudinal studies. It appears to me that Shalev's key constructs, such as pretraumatic heightened reactivity, heightened conditionability, and impaired extinction, are strongly linked to cognitive-affective units because personality risk factors might also be expressed psychophysiologically. For example, "neuroticism/negative emotionality," which Schnurr and Vielhauer propose as a likely risk factor for PTSD, is a multifaceted construct that includes psychophysiological components such as heightened reactivity to stress, oversensitivity to negative events, negativistic appraisal, and emotional lability (Watson et al. 1994). Furthermore, the psychophysiological abnormalities in reactivity, conditionability, and extinction will probably affect personality variables as expressed by cognitive-affective units such as encoding, expectancies and beliefs, and affects. Rigorous, hypothesis-driven, multimodal, and multidisciplinary research will be required before we can understand how each specific risk factor for PTSD simultaneously affects cognitive, emotional, behavioral, psychophysiological, and psychobiological processes. I believe that this is a very exciting and relevant future direction for research in this area.

Finally, McFarlane synthesizes much of this material by focusing on the capacity of an acutely traumatized individual "to modulate his or her acute stress response and to restore psychological and biological homeostasis" as one of the best indicators of vulnerability to, or protection from, subsequent development of PTSD (see Chapter 8). Experiential, familial, cognitive, psychological, and biological risk factors may all adversely affect the post-traumatic transitional state, when the immediate adaptive challenge is resolution of the acute stress response. Inability to cope with this challenge may lead to PTSD. Prompt detection and intervention, on the other hand, may lead to a more favorable outcome. Indeed, McFarlane's comprehensive model acknowledges the complexity of PTSD and identifies many different points of potential vulnerability, each of which may hamper the capacity to cope with a traumatic event. It is a very good place to begin as we develop proactive strategies to forestall the later development of PTSD, especially among those at greatest risk.

Future Research

All scientific knowledge can be misused. In the case of risk factors for PTSD, a worst-case scenario would be to exclude people from certain careers because they happen to be female or to have a family history of depression or to possess any other characteristic correlated with vulnerability to PTSD. I will not belabor the point that most of our current information is cross-sectional, is based on very few studies, has not established causality, and has only begun to help us understand etiology.

A best-case scenario is to amplify the momentum generated by the work described in this book and to aggressively explicate the mechanisms through which risk factors express themselves with respect to PTSD symptomatology. Next, we should seek to develop interventions that might normalize dysfunctional cognitive-affective units, abnormal psychophysiological responses, or alterations in other relevant etiological processes. In the same way that physicians have learned to prescribe protective dietary and behavioral strategies for people at risk for cardiovascular disease or cancer, we must strive to discover psychological, psychophysiological, and psychobiological strategies that will fortify resistance and reduce vulnerability, especially among individuals who are at the greatest risk for developing PTSD.

References

American Psychiatric Association: Diagnostic and Statistical Manual of Mental Disorders, 3rd Edition. Washington, DC, American Psychiatric Association, 1980

American Psychiatric Association: Diagnostic and Statistical Manual of Mental Disorders, 4th Edition. Washington, DC, American Psychiatric Association, 1994

Foa EB, Steketee G, Rothbaum BO: Behavioral/cognitive conceptualizations of posttraumatic stress disorder. Behavior Therapy 20:155–176, 1989

Friedman M, Charney DS, Deutch AY: Neurobiological and Clinical Consequences of Stress: From Normal Adaptation to Post-Traumatic Stress Disorder. Philadelphia, PA, Lippincott–Raven, 1995

Griffin SJ, Friedman MF: Depressive symptoms in propranolol users. J Clin Psychiatry 47:453–457, 1986

Mischel W, Shoda Y: A cognitive-affective system theory of personality: reconceptualizing situations, dispositions, dynamics, and invariance in personality structure. Psychol Rev 102:246–268, 1995

Watson D, Clark LS, Harkness AR: Structures of personality and their relevance to psychopathology. J Abnorm Psychol 103:18–31, 1994

Yehuda R, McFarlane AC: Conflict between knowledge about posttraumatic stress disorder and its original conceptual basis. Am J Psychiatry 152:1705–1713, 1995

Index

*Page numbers printed in **boldface** type refer to tables or figures.*

variations of in studies using DSM-III criteria, 24–25

Prisoners-of-war (POW), and dose-response model of stress and risk of PTSD, 7

Project TALENT, 211

Propranolol, and depression scores on Hamilton Depression Scale, 225

Protective factor. *See* Risk factors

Psychophysiological research, on risk factors for PTSD
definitions of relevant terms, 143–144
etiology and, 157–158
findings of, 149–157
measures used in, 144–149

PTSD. *See* Posttraumatic stress disorder

Race, and prevalence of PTSD in National Comorbidity Survey, **38**, 41, 43–44

Randomly selected traumas. *See also* Trauma and traumatic events
genetic and family environment and risk of experiencing, 71–72
National Comorbidity Survey and, 50, 52–54

Rape. *See also* Sexual abuse; Sexual assault
cortisol levels in victims of, 178
differential risk of PTSD by trauma type in National Comorbidity Survey, 31, 35, 52

exposure scale for intensity of as traumatic stressor, 8

family studies of PTSD and, 87, 88

interviews and research methodology, 29–30

Reactivity, and psychophysiological studies, 145–146

Recent Life Events Scale, 113

Reexperiencing symptoms, and PTSD
genetic and environmental factors in, 74
level of combat exposure and, **68**, 69

Regions (of United States), and prevalence of PTSD in National Comorbidity Survey, **39**, 43

Rehearsal, and psychophysiological studies on PTSD, 146–147

Research. *See also* Posttraumatic stress disorder; Risk factors
design of
archival studies, 16
cross-sectional epidemiological studies, 17
family studies, 17
genetic studies, 17–18, 62–63
longitudinal studies, 18–20
twin studies, 64–66
influence on revision of diagnostic criteria for PTSD in DSMs, 24, 168

interviews and research
methodology, 29–30
neurological soft signs in
women with PTSD
resulting from, 130
studies of adult children of
Holocaust survivors and,
95
Sexual assault, and dose-response
model of relationship between
stress and risk of PTSD, 7. *See
also* Rape; Physical assault;
Sexual abuse
Shell shock
family history of
psychoneurosis and, 81,
88
history of concepts of acute
stress disorders, 169
Shipley Institute of Living Scale,
129
Skin conductance habituation, in
trauma survivors and PTSD
patients, 155–156, 157
Sleep, difficulty with as symptom
of posttraumatic stress
disorder, 74
Social functioning, and acute stress
disorders in combat veterans,
171. *See also* Personal
relationships
Somatic symptoms, and
combat-related stress, 171
Specificity, of family history in
studies of PTSD, 85
Spiegel, J. P., 170
Startle
proneness as symptom of PTSD
and genetic studies, 87

psychophysiological studies
of PTSD and, 147,
154–157
Stress and stressors. *See also*
Acute stress disorders;
Trauma and traumatic
events
acute vs. chronic reactions to,
11
adult children of Holocaust
survivors and, 103,
114–119
animal models for biological
response to, 177
discrimination of correlates of
PTSD from effects of
specific, 11–13
hippocampal volume and,
132–133
psychophysiological findings
in studies of PTSD and,
149–150
stress-diathesis model of
PTSD and characteristics
of, 6–9
Stress-diathesis model
of depression, 5, 225
role of personality in etiology
of PTSD and, 214,
216
as strategy for study of
development of PTSD,
4–11, 20
Stress-induced oscillation, and
future research on acute
stress response, 183
Structured Clinical Interview for
DSM-III, 113
Structured Clinical Interview for
DSM-III-R, 30, 127, 212